y beautiful
friend, Suzy x
Hope you enjoy.
Love Heather
xxx

Being Omni

Being Omni

Cover design by Zoë Gower-Jones
Illustrated by Heather Light

First printing, June 2018
Printed in Caerphilly, Wales by Horizon Digital Media Ltd.

ISBN 978-1-5272-2391-2

Being Omni

Simple steps to becoming you

Robert and Heather Light

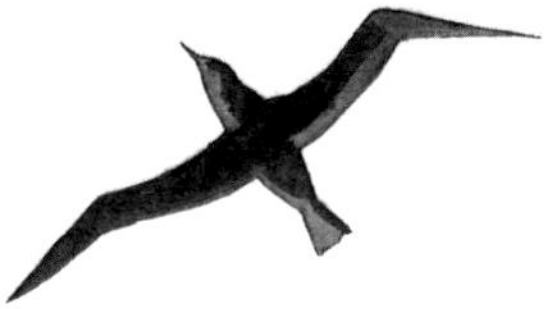

"You need to keep finding yourself,
a little more each day,
that real unlimited [human being].
He's your instructor."

Jonathan Livingston Seagull ~ Richard Bach

For
Yvonne
Becci
Jamie
&
Clare

Contents

A Proviso

Omni is guaranteed to work!
No ifs and buts – it works.
If you have been searching for answers,
the place to find them is within.
As you go through the book and start
to use the steps on a daily basis,
you will begin to notice changes within yourself
and the world around you.
The proviso is
that you use the three
Omni steps
at least 2 to 5 times, every day.
As you do, your life begins to improve.
Your body begins its natural healing process.
You become whole.
You begin to live rather than exist.
Omni cannot be used to change others.
They change automatically because you have changed.
With Omni, everyone you know or encounter will benefit
without you having to do anything.
If you use the three Omni steps daily,
life gets better and so do
YOU.

Opening Doors

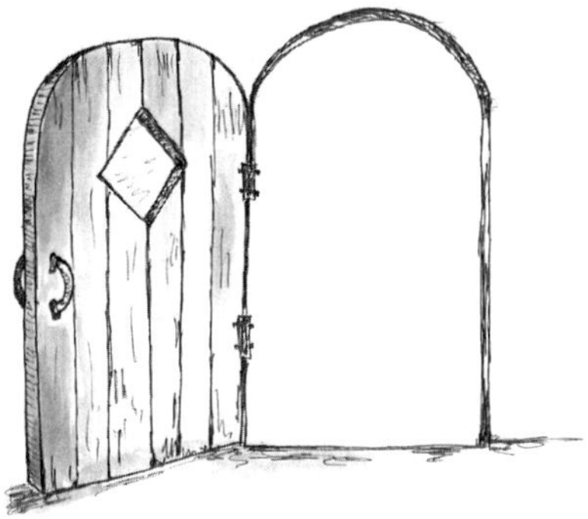

Everyone knows introductions serve a particular purpose and are usually brief and succinct, outlining or detailing the information that follows in the book. But this introduction is quite different. It is a working, *doing-as-you-read* introduction and this exactly as you should go with the rest of the book.

Being Omni is based around three simple steps. Congratulations, by the way, for taking the first step in buying this book and beginning to read it. And, as you practise the first few steps at least 3 to 5 times daily, change within will begin to happen.

We often avoid change, even fear it at times. When anyone mentions things changing, it can start off a chain of thoughts and one of them is usually believing it's going to require some kind of enormous effort. An effort we are obviously far, far too busy for and we end up convincing ourselves that things are fine the way they are. But what if there was a way to create change and flow and movement within your life without very much effort at all? A way that is simple and straightforward. A way that will make such a difference to your life and how you live and doesn't actually require any radical changes at all. If this sounds good, then this is just the book for you.

The Omni steps, which make up the core of this book, really do make change effortless. The secret here is that they take *thinking* out of the equation and just focus on *doing*. To take a step is an action and this will begin a natural process of change that requires minimal effort for really incredible, life-enhancing gains.

◊ STEP = you are doing something; an action instead of a thought.
◊ STEP = you move from a point of stuck-ness.
◊ STEP = you move to do something e.g. the breathing exercise.
◊ And because this book is laid out differently, you STEP out of the *known* into the *unknown*.

Of course, a lot depends on whether you will give the Omni steps a chance. You never know until you try. You can stay exactly the same, staying in the same routines, habits and old ways of living, or you can use Being Omni to start a process of self-betterment which not only helps you but everyone around you without much effort on your part at all.

The steps really will open the door to a new way of being and living your life.

Are you ready?

*****

Reference Points

We will start by creating some reference points. It's a good idea to have these as you go through this journey towards real and true freedom of yourself. These are your pre-Omni views of yourself so that you now have something you can look back on and compare with. Despite all of our advances in science and medicine, we have not as yet learnt to know ourselves. We think we know the image of ourselves but that actually comes via the mind. Your journey with Omni will help you become your true self and life then begins.

Ask yourself the following questions and please try and answer as honestly as you can. It will be of great benefit if you do.

- Are you happy and content with your life or is it just okay?
- Are there some aspects of your life that you would like to improve?
- How is your health and well-being?
- You have, after all, got this far in life, but does it live up to your expectations?
- Are your needs and wants fulfilled?
- Do you believe there is more to life and everyday living?

These questions are not meant to cause upset or distress but to get you to consider how you are living and experiencing life. After three to four weeks of using the Omni steps, please do a re-evaluation of yourself and your life and note any differences, no matter how big or small.

Let's have a go at the first step...

Step One

Breathing

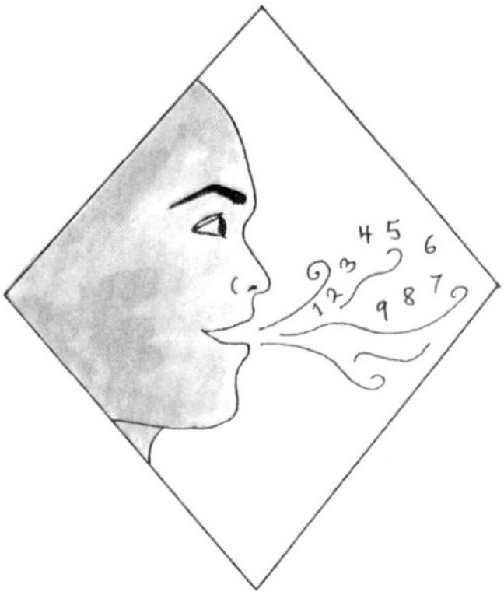

The first step in Being Omni is a breathing exercise. This particular exercise is all about taking *conscious control* of your breathing and in doing so, you begin to learn how to settle and quieten the mind (albeit temporarily). This has truly wonderful outcomes as it is guaranteed to give you some much needed space and respite AND it brings you into the present.

We've all heard about breathing exercises; they are age old techniques from many, many different cultures and practices around the world. However, this one is different. This one works because it becomes part of your living experience. Lots of breathing techniques ask us to find a quiet place and close our eyes. Although this might have its benefits, it really only ends up removing you from the reality of your experience. For this step, there is complete awareness of and focus on each phase of the breathing process allowing you to stay connected to your environment and increasing your general awareness.

Breathing is something that is usually regulated by your autonomic system within the cerebellum part of the brain, meaning it is not something we have to 'think' about; it happens automatically as part of our survival system. Here, you are taking over this autonomic system by controlling three stages: the length of your in-breath, how long you hold your breath (the pause) and a slow, controlled out-breath.

For this step to work effectively, we do not stick to a fixed number (e.g. breathe in for 5, hold for 5 and out for 5) but will use a random and irregular counting method. The reason for this is because the mind prefers routine and structure - and if you fall into a regular, rhythmic pattern of breathing, it is very easy for the mind and thoughts to take over again. By varying the breathing and by focusing on the counting, the mind doesn't drift as much. Your thoughts are brought into the present moments and you actually become more fully aware of your body and surroundings.

However, to start with, it is helpful to minimise distractions. It's also better if you are sitting or standing up rather than lying down and your eyes should remain open. This is not a meditative state as such but an active, fully awake and aware one. *Please remember that you should never try the breathing exercises whilst driving or operating machinery as you are increasing the amount of oxygen in your body.*

And breathe...

- o Make sure you are sitting up straight, shoulders back, with both feet on the floor and resting your hands comfortably on your thighs. Find your sitting bones[1] and ensure they are equal and balanced. You should feel relaxed while holding good posture - no slouching!
- o Now, use the following counting method: breathe in slowly for a count of 5, pause and hold your breath for a count of 7. Then breathe out, controlling the out-breath, for a count of 9. *(If 5 is too high, start with 3, 5, 7. The point is not to struggle or strain - basically you can create your own breathing count as long as it's random).*
- o Next, breathe in for 7, hold for 9 and breathe out for 11.
- o For each cycle of this controlled breathing, try a different combination of numbers: 7, 5, 9 - 5, 9, 7 - 9, 11, 7, for example. Try and stick to odd numbers too.
- o Allow yourself time to build up to longer cycles such as 13, 19, 27.
- o You are increasing the amount of oxygen in your body quite quickly here so go back to normal breathing if you become light-headed.

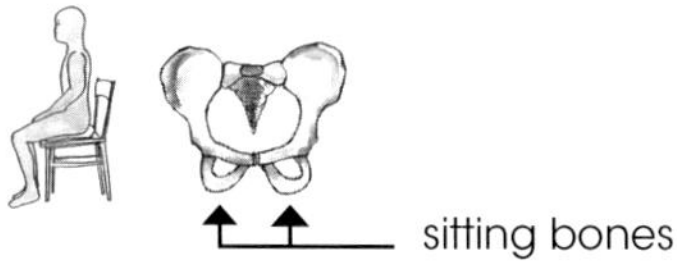

[1] Finding your sitting bones helps your posture, and you can gain anywhere from 1 – 1 ½" in height.

- This exercise requires you to do deep breathing or 'belly breathing'. If you haven't tried this before, you will notice the difference immediately. Most of us breathe in a very shallow way, with the chest and shoulders rising slightly. Deep breathing should reach the lower part of your lungs making your stomach expand. To check this, place one hand on your stomach and one on your chest. Breathe in slowly and allow your stomach to rise and expand as much as possible.
- To complete the cycle, the exhale is just as important. To achieve a longer out breath, you should try a slow, controlled exhalation where your stomach muscles contract as much as possible.
- Please try and repeat these random number counts between 5 to 8 times in one sitting (it should only take about five minutes) and a few times throughout the day. It fits well with a morning, noon and night cycle. You could set a timer on your phone as a reminder.
- This has to be done a few times throughout the day to realise the benefits of becoming you, becoming whole and moving into your correct time and space. This is especially important: the more you put into this step, the more time and space you will have.

Congratulations for practising the first step!

How did it go?

As you were counting, did your thoughts diminish? Did you feel more relaxed yet not sleepy? How about energised? How was your vision? It's a good idea now and again to look at a few things in the distance as you are adjusting your sitting bones and posture. Pick one or two things to focus on – I usually pick an ornament near the window and a tree or something outside in the distance. After the breathing exercise, my eyesight seems sharper and clearer and I can also see more detail in those things.

Journal opportunity ~ Keeping a record or note of how it went, how you felt before, during and after, will hopefully encourage you to keep practising. Have a think about how your day went. Did anything different happen? How did you react to others? Were you able to do the breathing at different times throughout the day? If not, why? What excuses did your mind conjure up to prevent this?

There is much out there on the benefits of breathing, especially deep and controlled breathing. It is a renowned technique to use during times of stress or panic and is also a brilliant re-set method. See the chapters on *The Benefits of Breathing* and *Re-set Methods* for more details.

> *"For me, I really make a point of sitting tall on my sitting bones and aligning myself as best I can, feeling my feet to assist a more balanced energy flow. After some while*

of practising, it is surprising how few slow, controlled breaths are needed. Maybe even three rounds can be enough to make a difference. I am no expert at holding my breath or making a long count but it seems the pause is most important and somehow it works."

Jenny Underhill

Ways to use your journal

Lots of people write a journal or keep a diary of events and experiences in their lives. This is good but it also stores our emotional responses and our hurts alongside our joys and wonders. When we look back over the journal, we remember and we **still** *feel and respond to these events as ourselves at that time, not the self we are today. Of course, our memories of events are also triggered randomly, but it has the same effect. We react or respond to these from that specific point in time. Photographs cause a smile or frown at times too.*

For your Omni journey, a new type of journal is much needed. So, we obtain an A4 booklet that is worthy of this great work!

Once you have one, go to the middle and write today's date and then just jot down a few things that are happening and how you are feeling at this time. Next, go to the first page and write your full name, the date and time you were born, the place where you were born (which gives you your star sign and a numerological number too), and add your parents' names in full.

The next page is for your first birthday, the following for your second birthday and so on right up to your present age where you have written the current date (if you are as old as me I had to go near the back of book to write the present day in).

As and when, aim to jot down little memories on the age pages as they fit. Keep doing this every so often and your life story will soon become history that has less and less impact on your present moments.

Living or Existing

This stage of your Omni journey is all about putting yourself first and allowing you to focus on you for a change. This is *your* personal journey to self-discovery and self-betterment and self-mastery and self-awareness. See – self, self, self! And because this stage is all about doing something, it will be of great benefit to you if you practise the steps daily.

As you step into the Being Omni world, things within you change and so do the connections and contacts in your external world. This happens because you start to *be in* Omni. The state of existing, becomes a statement of actual change (*being* becomes *be in*), and there is a world of difference between existing and living.

The three very simple steps really will begin to alter and improve your state of being. This simply means the way you *live* and experience your life ~ it's about how you think and what you do, how you react and respond to the different people and situations in your life and, most importantly, how you feel about yourself.

> *"Before I started this journey, although I was relatively happy, I felt like life was just happening to me and I*

had very little control. The pace of my life seemed to be speeding up and I was becoming stressed and anxious. I had more and more things on my plate and seemingly less and less time to do anything. I felt like I was just existing."

Heather Light

This current state of existing is how others have often described their lives and how things are going for them. And we can go on living this way for years. For many of us, this way of life has become the norm.

◊ *Presently, life has become about existing rather than living. No matter where you are, life around you has been getting faster and faster and faster. Time seems to get swallowed up. Being Omni will help you begin to live again and put the brakes on the hamster wheel. It will also give you more actual, real time to enjoy your life once more.*

Of course, this is not to say that you are unhappy. You might be perfectly content with the way you are living and experiencing your life, but this doesn't mean the Omni steps can't help you too. Whether you are happy and enjoying life or at the very least feel there is an imbalance with the way you live, try them and see if life gets better for you.

One of the main reasons this type of existing happens is because we are at the mercy of our minds and are at a point where our thoughts and how we think, dominate. There is more and more research out there which scientifically proves how much time we spend thinking. A recent Harvard study[2] claims we spend 43% of our time thinking. I would say that it feels more like 90%.

Too much thinking and being overwhelmed by thoughts is something many of us would like to change. We would like to change this because when our thoughts are seemingly endless and we are unable to control them or stop them or even just switch off for a bit, it can leave us feeling powerless. Just think about how many thoughts you can have in an hour! Thoughts about what you should be doing, what you have to do, what you haven't done, replaying the day's events and interactions, over-analysing anything and everything, and jumping around from the past to imagining future events, is a familiar experience for many of us.

To put this into visual perspective, the following image represents how the majority of us are living today. We spend most of our time in the mind. The head is so out of proportion to the body to show how we spend a large amount of time thinking.

[2] The Harvard Gazette, 'Wandering mind not a happy mind', Steve Bradt, November 2010.

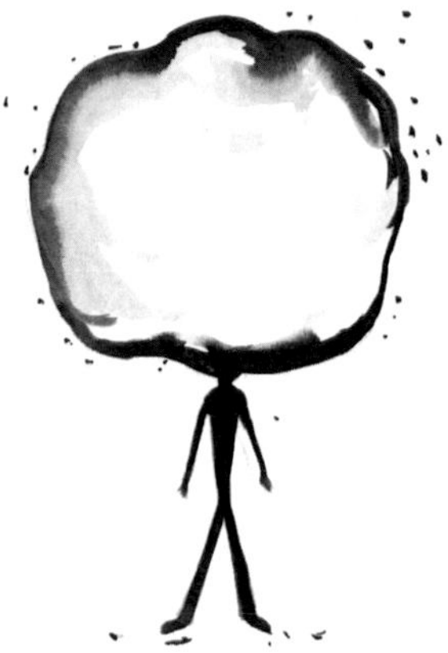

By introducing the three very simple steps into your life, it can immediately give you a sense of control and balance back. The steps will show you how to get less bombarded by your thoughts and, perhaps for the first time ever, you are doing something that make the mind and all the thinking take a back seat.

As you can probably tell by now, in essence, Being Omni is all about *doing*. And doing rather than thinking of doing are two very different things. It sounds obvious but if you are actually doing something (practising the steps), it triggers a whole set of behind-the-scenes responses because basically you are giving yourself the message that you are worth doing something for. You are taking steps which show a commitment to improving yourself and the way you are living and experiencing your life.

Most importantly, the steps are all *internally* orientated. This means the focus is on the body and the senses. By concentrating on what you *feel*, you begin to reduce all the mind noise and learn to begin to develop a much better connection to your body and your true self. It's like making friends with yourself at last.

◊ *Each of the steps move you into a state of being and a state of doing – for the two go hand in hand. It is a true state of internal change which in turn will affect your external world. You could liken it to meditation in the sense that, while practising, the feelings of balance and harmony may only last a while, but your ability to go in and out of Being Omni begins to have a lasting effect. All this requires is commitment from you, for you.*

*****

Controlled Breathing ~ A closer look

At first, you may feel like nothing is happening or that you don't feel any different, but this is what's actually happening...

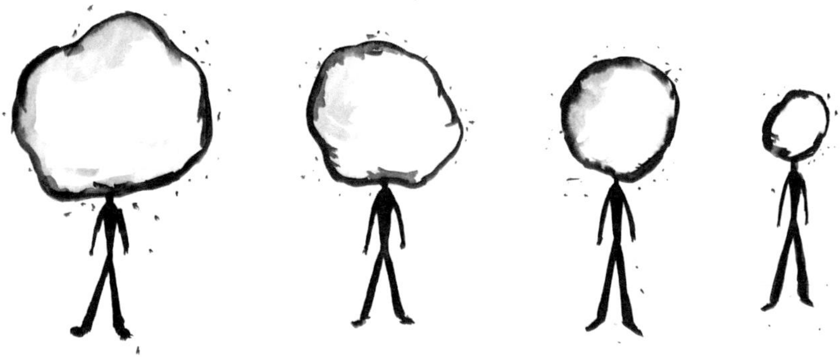

As you practise this step throughout the day, you can see that with each image the size of the head reduces. Each time you complete a breathing cycle it addresses this imbalance as the only purpose for your thoughts is to work with you as you breathe. Hence, they become more manageable and less unruly.

It brings your thoughts more inside where, instead of being about the past or future, they are more in the here and nows.

◊ *Nows may seem like a funny word and grammatically incorrect; however, by creating a plural form of now it allows us flexibility in the moment. The present is not a fixed time. It is constantly moving. Accordingly, an awareness of the words we use to describe things is important: how you think, what you say, how you say it, all has an effect. As we adapt our language, so do the connotations attached to it adapt so they are more suitable. Breaking a few rules of grammar is allowed on your Omni journey!*

The more you practise, the more it reduces the amount of thinking you do and you will get less battered by your thoughts and become more balanced and whole in the process. As you become less bombarded you should also begin to experience fewer thoughts. As soon as you have fewer thoughts or less thinking, something amazing happens ~ you begin to have more actual space and time for you.

◊ *Less thinking = more you.*

*****

Less is More

Less is More is an active principle and fundamental to Being Omni. It refers to how much a person lives or exists from their mind's view of *everything* and how, by using the steps, we can begin to shift away from this.

When the mind gets in the way, it actually prevents us from doing things. We over-think, over-analyse, get into all sorts of knots and usually end up doing nothing.

Thinking is the antagonist of doing!

The Omni steps are designed so that we use less of the mind to achieve them because they are *doing* things. The reason the breathing step requires randomness is because the mind likes order and uniformity and when something is contrary to this, it disengages somewhat from what you are doing so we have less mind, so to speak, and more doing. You are able to switch off this autonomic part of your brain by using your mind to create a set of thoughts (the breathing count) which you then turn into an action.

Less is more seems a bit of contradictory statement but nevertheless, once you enter the Omni world, it becomes truer.

It becomes truer because the Omni steps help us have fewer thoughts. And when you start Being Omni and move more and more into real time and nows, those thoughts slip into your history files and *no longer drive decisions you make*. The amount of space you used to take up before Omni was very large. Being Omni reduces this dramatically so less is more: less mind equals more you, more time and more space to be in.

Once you introduce the first few steps into your daily lives, you will be astounded at how your world responds...so don't just read, do. See for yourself.

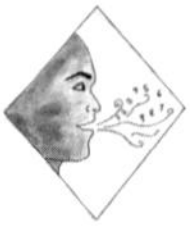

Pause for a moment and try the breathing step again, right now, please.

*****

The Benefits of Breathing

At any point during the day, try and pay attention to how you breathe – if it's shallow, then switch to deep. And if you need any more encouragement, just look at all the other well-known benefits!

Deep breathing...

- o makes you calmer
- o increases oxygen in the body
- o helps to detoxify the body
- o relieves pain
- o stimulates the lymphatic system

o increases our cardiovascular capacity
o gives you energy
o helps your digestion
o strengthens the major organs

Deep breathing is one of the easiest ways to improve your overall health and is something that you can do anywhere, at any time. It costs nothing and takes very little effort. Take a little time each day to practise and your efforts will be greatly rewarded.

> *"Applying the simple and relaxing Omni steps with consistency and dedication brought about such changes in me. From barely existing within a spiral of anxiety, doubt, fear and pain, to a feeling of being 'freed' and awakened to the potential in all of my living moments. I am now living with confidence, strength and an inner peace - with a deep sense of awareness and well-being. I feel less affected, dependent on or hurt by others' approval, love or opinions. There are many ways revealed to us on our life's journey. Being Omni is a gateway, a path of self-discovery, not tied to any belief or religion which brings improvement to my state of living and being - a gift to humanity which I feel extremely privileged to have had revealed to me."*

Amanda D Carter

*****

Further Practice with Step One

As you practise this step you won't necessarily have to seek a quiet environment. The better you get, you will find that you can do the breathing step when you're out and about. Experimenting is the key here as it is about integrating the steps into your everyday lives and situations.

You're constantly interacting with different people, places and things; therefore, it is not always about the peace and quiet but engaging with your surroundings. Becoming more aware of how you interact, how different places and situations affect you, gives you a chance to notice how these interactions are enhanced when you practise the steps.

Try controlled breathing in different locations: a park; a busy shopping centre; under a tree; on a beach; by flowing water or the place where you work. Pay attention to how you respond to your immediate environment, be it a busy or a quiet one. When you're doing the breathing exercise, does anything change?

Living in the Present

Another aspect of our lives too much thinking affects, is the ability to access or live in the present. Existing in our thoughts, living in the mind, pretty much guarantees we end up paying little or no attention to it.

Well, in all honesty, due to the current way we live and experience our lives, the present often *is* unreachable. Everyone these days is talking about it, and explaining that we should all live in the present and that this is the best way to be, but how do you know when you are in the present? How do you actually do this – live in the present? There are countless self-help books out there that claim to teach us how, but it can still seem like some never-never land. It's perhaps helpful to admit that, for the majority of us, it *is* difficult to live in the present.

The good news is, the Omni steps provide a way to access the present, and not just any present either, your present. They can show you how to experience it so you become more aware of living in your present. The more you practise the steps, the easier this becomes. In fact, it becomes automatic and natural. As the steps are integrated into your daily life, the more you can have longer, more sustained experiences of being and living in the reality of your present flowing moments ~ and the benefits of this are incredible.

- o Your health improves because the Omni steps bring to the fore your inherent self-healing abilities.
- o You acquire more energy because living presently has the least detrimental impact to you and everything around you. There is less impact on you, the world and the people around you.
- o You are flowing in real time, not mind time.
- o You have fewer thoughts because you are not in mind time.
- o You experience more connection as you are increasing your awareness ~ firstly for yourself, then for others and finally the world around you.
- o You become a shining example to others. People will wonder why you look so vibrant.
- o The ups and downs of everyday living are more in balance.
- o You begin to establish a greater rapport with every other living thing.
- o There is much less time being annoyed or angry or down.

> *"I first discovered Omni when I went along to a presentation in 2015. At that time, my health and confidence were at a low ebb. I'm so pleased I made this choice, otherwise my life would not have changed. I learnt that by focusing on the breath I got a sense of how my body felt in that moment. By using the breathing to be in my moments, it stopped me thinking*

of past or future events and when I concentrated on being present in my moments, I actually enjoyed them! It gave me a space that allowed the freedom to just be. Being Omni is helping me break free from my self-made imprisonment and I am very grateful to the Omni team. The journey for me has been amazing. It has helped me discover myself. Instead of Wo[3] and baggage which is full of emotions, I present myself as Sandra Davies."

Sandra Davies

*****

Health and well-being

It might be difficult to believe that a simple breathing exercise can actively benefit your health and well-being but it's true. We can no longer ignore, as more and more research is finally beginning to acknowledge and prove, the direct correlation between our well-being state and our health. Of course, there are many other factors involved: what you eat and drink, whether you do any exercise, where you live and so on. To have a fully active life, you need to be fit and healthy for sure, but many modern illnesses are very much to do with the mind and how stress, anxiety and depression can and do cause illnesses. According to MIND, one in four people will experience mental health issues.[4] It is endemic in our current society, and we

[3] Wo is a character from the collection of parables by Lee Carroll, The Parables of Kryon (Kyron Series)

[4] www.mind.org.uk – Mental health facts and statistics

have reached a crisis point. The body suffers the ravages of the mind and there is now a growing awareness of what stress does to our health. More importantly, once this is recognised we can begin to learn and experience that we are absolutely NOT powerless in this situation.

In many Eastern medicines, philosophies and practices, the teaching encourages you to become proactive so the onus is on the person. Looking for prevention rather than cure is very much the individual's responsibility. Whereas in the West, there is more emphasis on seeking outside for help and on focusing on the cure. For many, this has stopped us learning how to trust and listen to ourselves. Of course, orthodox medicine is absolutely necessary but that doesn't mean we can't do more to help ourselves too.

This journey is about many things but one of the most important is learning that you can actively make a huge difference to your health and well-being and a good place to start is following these simple steps. By *doing* something you grow and change, but by *thinking* something nothing much happens. This is why implementing and doing the steps will cause a radical shift in consciousness which in turn will improve your everyday health and living.

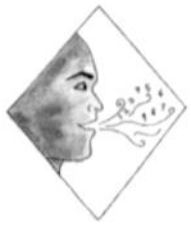

Pause and take a moment to do Step One again before we move on.

Mind and Body

Out of the three Omni steps, Step Two is the one that will make the biggest difference. The main purpose is re-connecting the mind to the body so we begin to function as the one unit we are supposed to be.

Connecting the mind to the body may sound a bit strange as, obviously, the head is joined to the body but really most of us are totally unaware of our bodies. Think about the times that you do pay attention to your body. Is it only when something is wrong? Or when you have pain or discomfort? Is it when you are not happy about the way your body might look? Does your body have to fit the modern-day criteria of how it should look?

We have grown separate from ourselves because we dwell mostly in our thoughts which are never in the reality of the moments. This means that the mind and body have also become separated.

The main focus of Step One is to help with a busy mind by bringing your thoughts more into the body where they become more internalised by focusing on your breathing. This is difficult if not impossible to do when your thoughts are anywhere and everywhere. This is why practising controlled breathing a few times throughout the day will really help before you move onto this next one. Step Two builds on this and takes us through how to begin connecting your mind and thoughts to your body. By developing a relationship with and connection to your wonderful body, you not only begin to live more presently but you begin to learn a whole new language.

Journal opportunity ~ Make a note of your answers to the following questions and please be as honest as you can. How often do you notice or listen to your body? Do you even know how?

Step Two is all about learning how our thoughts can actually be quite useful when we begin to *consciously direct* and *control* them. And rather than the ongoing, typical negative dialogue we have about our bodies, we are going to use our thoughts to establish a connection between mind and body that will benefit you in so many ways.

Using the mind, you are going to send a thought to an area of your body. All this means is for you to first think about a part of your body. At this point, you might be wondering 'And?' as it seems like nothing much happens, but let's explore this process.

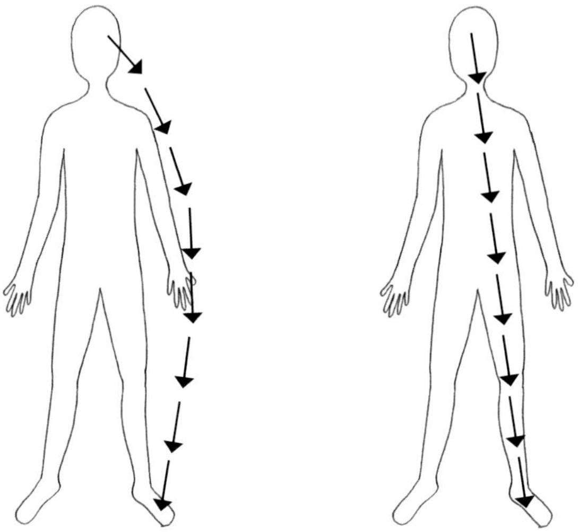

If your thoughts travel externally, like the first image, then you end up with a mind-based response. A standard, default response like 'Fine' or 'Okay'. As you can see, your thoughts bypass your body completely. However, if we bring the thoughts in and connect to our nervous system via our senses, then you are connecting to your body. Your thoughts move through your body to the area you are focusing on as the second image depicts. We can check this is happening by being able to pick up different sensory information. This is a truly incredible shift as it is the beginning of accessing your senses and using them inwards.

◊ *Thinking about something = nothing much happens, but when the thought connects to a part of your body, your body communicates back via sensations and so begins a new language.*

This new language is the language of the body which is vastly different from the mind's dialogue. Why? Because the mind is conditioned and your thoughts are a mixture of different times (past, present, future) whereas the body is actually existing in the present. This will be explained in more detail as we go, but for now to begin to experience this we will focus on the five external senses: see, hear, touch, taste and smell.

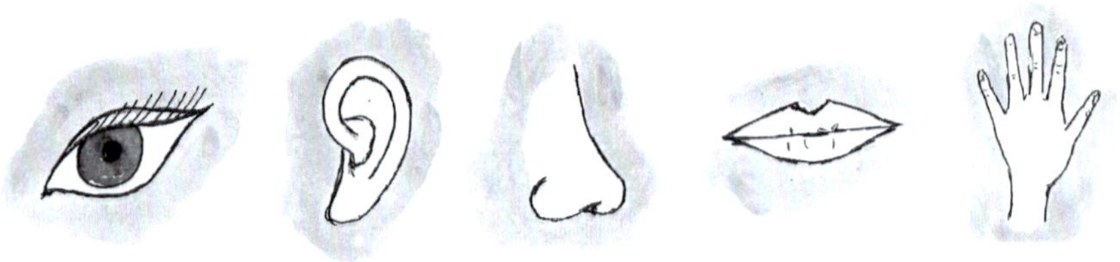

The senses are one of the body's ways of communicating to you via the nervous system where they are immediately sending messages back and forth to the brain, all synapses firing. Once we have this information (e.g. heat – pain – hard surface), there are various ways we interpret it which leads to a reaction or response.

◊ *Working with the basics of what we all know and understand, your body via your senses is directly linked to the present, to your immediate surroundings and situation.*

I know it seems obvious but say, for example, when you are sat working at the computer, how much attention do you pay to your weight on the chair? Or your fingers tapping away at the keyboard and the sounds happening all around you? How much of your focus is actually on these things? Often, we are so caught up in what we are doing, we pay very little attention indeed.

Let's see if we can change this by having a go at Step Two.

∞

Step Two

Feeling and Sensing

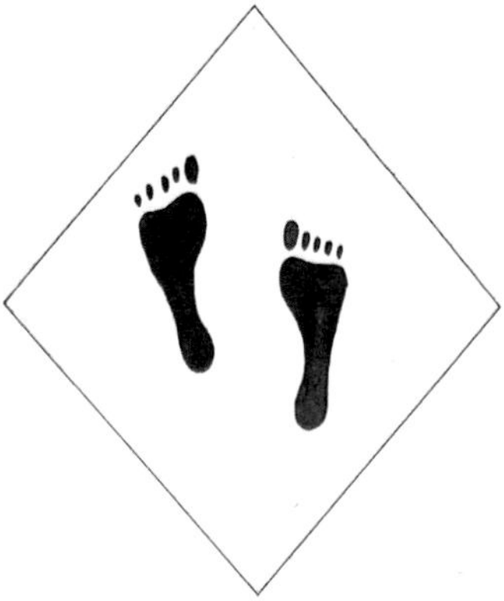

Again, we will start will some basic questions.

How are your feet? How do they feel?

These may seem like funny questions to start with, but what are your answers? Did you look at your feet when you were thinking about them? Perhaps they don't 'feel' anything at all.

We start with the feet because they are the body part which is the furthest from our heads. They carry us around all day long, bearing the weight of the body but are often neglected and hardly ever thought about...unless there's a problem.

These two questions have been the starting point of many talks and courses over the years and all sorts of answers appear.

Most people tend to actually look down at them – yes, they are there, attached to your legs! Then the verbal response will be, 'Fine, thank you' or 'Okay'.

These are 'mind-based' responses.

Just think about when someone asks how you are. There is no detail or truth, just an automatic, conditioned response. It's probably our default response for any number of reasons at the time, but for this step, learning how to recognise when you slip into a mind-based response rather than a body one, will be of great benefit in helping you to master this step...and it is a big step.

So, what we really want is how they *feel*. After practice, this should elicit a difference set of internal physical sensory responses such as:

✓ Heavy or light
✓ Achy
✓ Warm or cool

It truly is one of the most exciting and incredible shifts when you begin to reconnect to your body and are able to focus on the physical (sensory) and immediate information it gives you. This forgotten way of communicating certainly is like learning a new language and provides a point from which so much can happen: self-healing, a quieter mind, accessing your truths, taking up less space, living in the moments...the list goes on and on. These first two steps really can make a difference.

Let's give it a go...

How do your feet feel?

This may seem hard work or strange to begin with but please persevere, and to minimise the mind's interference your feet will either be light or heavy, warm or cold so check and sense and feel how your feet are right now. You might find it easier to just focus on one, your right or left. You could be sitting there for a while thinking, they don't feel anything. Try then to focus on a specific part of the foot. For example, the soles of your feet. All your attention and focus go here. If your mind wanders, put your attention back on this area until you begin to *feel* something. It could be a niggle or tingling. It could be a real sense of temperature. Once you can elicit something like this, you now have something to work with and it's much easier to keep focusing on this area.

◊ *REMEMBER - right now is the only time that truly exists, everything else exists only within the mind. Your body exists in real time...the mind does not, therefore, your body is the key to accessing the reality of the present.*

Let's say one foot feels warm and heavy, are both feet the same warmth? Are they exactly the same weight? This is referring to their weight on the floor. Check again and slowly but surely see if they will begin to match up.

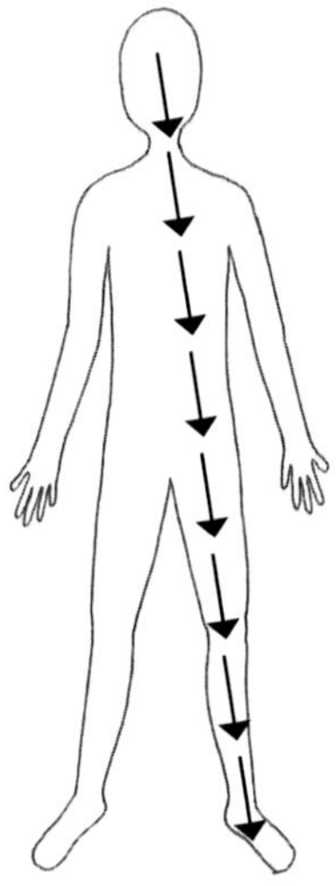

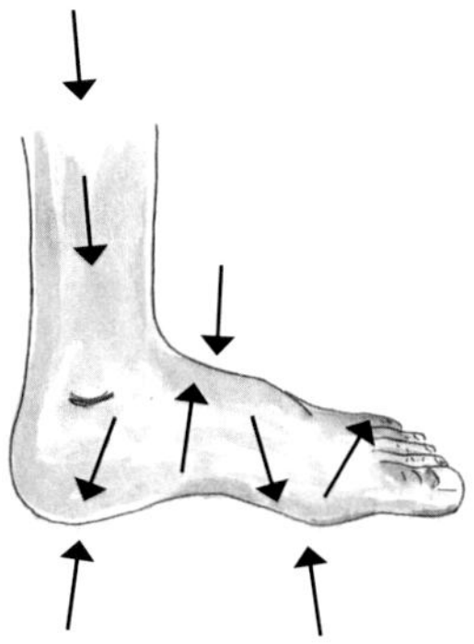

As you begin to think 'How are my feet?', a set of signals travel down through your body (remember there is a difference with your thoughts travelling externally to internally) until they reach your feet, and the sensory answer or response flows back to your mind. The picture of the foot depicts both the external and the internal information. You can determine whether your thoughts are travelling internally through your body by picking up this sensory information.

However, because we are not used to keeping our minds focused on one particular area or thing, our thoughts easily try and distract us in any way that they can.

Stick with it.

Let your thoughts come and go then put your attention back on your feet. If you can sense weight or temperature, then this is a truly great start.

Once you are able to sense this, and keep awareness of this feeling, it is around this point that a sensation of tingling (like pins and needles) should begin to happen: this is the nervous system waking up under conscious control.

Keep focusing on the tingling or pulsing feeling, something you might never have been aware of or experienced before, but you are using your sense of touch inwards and now have a rapport with your internal world of energy which can communicate information to you through the senses.

This is a reality.

Experiencing the pins and needles feelings is the first time that mind and body are at one. With practice, you can expand this tingling to the whole of your foot, then perhaps both feet. As you put your attention on your shins or calves, the tingling should begin to travel up your leg and appear here as well. You might lose the sensation in your feet but as soon as you focus back on them, looking for a physical sensation or reaction, it comes back. The aim is to be able to connect quickly where sensory communication restarts pretty much immediately.

Once you have a sense of tingling or whatever sensation in your feet, this becomes a message via your nervous system as a nerve line goes a short way then connects via a node point with many other nerve line signals. Your foot's feeling message goes onto the next node and finally into your brain to the receptors. The thought 'How are my feet?', then travels high speed back and forth and now you have a real connection.

As the signal flashes along your nerve lines and the tingles have begun, another system then comes into play called the meridian energy system. Here your mind and body connection allow the energy part to synchronise with your physical body.

You may or may not be aware of your energy counterpart. It might be something you are learning about or are completely and utterly sceptical of. It is certainly more challenging to accept when you are just reading about it – it is, however, something you can experience.

The Being Omni steps are all about bringing the mind, body and energy part together. When we have these three systems harmonised and working together in synchronicity, we become whole.

◊ *As we proceed, we shift from purely mind answers into the self's answers then slowly but surely into whole being answers.*

There is a chapter called, *Understanding Energy*, which has a more comprehensive explanation of the energy part and system.

Journal opportunity ~ Write about your first experience of this. Did it work? What did you notice?

As with Step One, begin to incorporate this into your daily routines, but try not to have fixed times or parameters. You will find that both of these steps are incredibly useful during moments throughout the day, say when something rattles you, or you get angry or hurt or are tired or overwhelmed.

*****

The Body and Real Time

Practising Step Two really does help you experience and live more in the present moments because the body is in real time. This means that it can *only* ever be in the present moment. Real time is actual, true time.

Rarely do we experience real time because our thoughts tend to favour the past or future. When your thoughts drift off (and this can be just thinking about something that happened yesterday or thinking ahead about what to have for dinner), it prevents us from being in the present. Your thoughts take you away from real time and because of this the mind and body are no longer connected: one is experiencing real time whereas the other is not and this means you are not working as a whole unit.

We can see the difference between your body being in real time as opposed to mind time if we have a look at a visual impact of thoughts.

Imagine thoughts are attached to you by an elastic thread. When we have a thought or bring a thought into existence, it doesn't just drift off and disappear. It is your thought and it is attached to you. Say for example, the thought about what you want to eat for dinner. That thought is in a future time, a time that doesn't even exist yet. It travels off to this future event and there is an actual pull or effect on the body. This pull happens because there is conflict – your thought is in one time and your body in another. When mind and body are one, acting as a whole unit, both are in real time and your body is no longer stretched and ravaged by your thoughts.

Take a look at the following image. The spikes and points are visual representations of thoughts, both emanating from the body and those exchanges from known or unknown external sources.

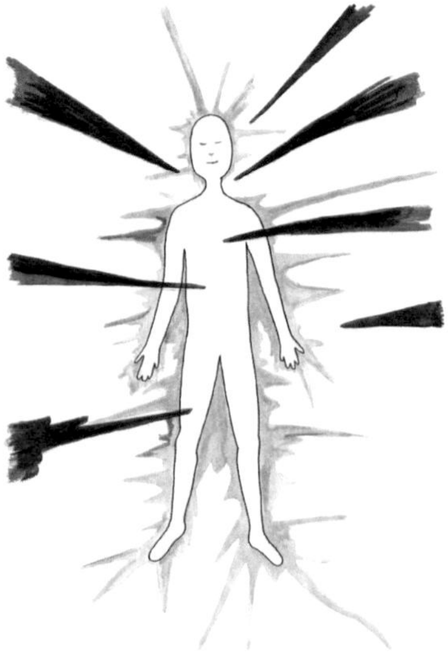

Compare this to image where the mind, body and energy part are as one. Here you are balanced and whole.

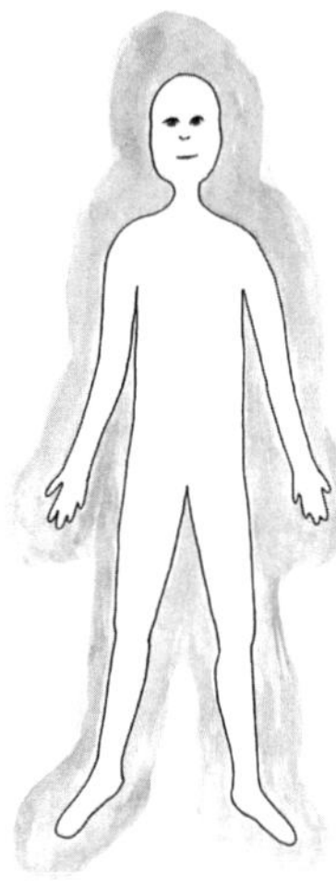

Step Two can help us address this and this truly is where the everyday magic can start to happen!

Step Two and Self-Healing

◊ *The Omni steps begin to awaken our innate but often forgotten abilities.*

One of the most significant and profoundly beneficial aspects of this step is that it brings to the fore our inherent ability to self-heal.

Your body truly is an amazing thing. It has the capabilities of self-healing, rejuvenation and regeneration and much more once the mind is no longer causing it problems. But due to the way we currently live, we use these self-healing abilities less and less. So much so, that the even idea of self-healing is alien or strange to some of us – or we simply don't even believe it is possible.

To keep this in perspective, there are things that happen in the everyday that testify to such abilities yet we still choose to ignore or disregard them. The idea that human beings are capable of self-healing or healing others is one of these. But by simply looking to the biology of the body we can see that it is a self-healing mechanism which constantly maintains and restores itself. Think about cuts or bruises, for example, and how they heal or how the liver is able to replace damaged tissue with new cells.

An obvious example to use here is when you have bumped into something or fallen over. What is the first thing you usually do to the area experiencing the most pain? You cover it with your hands. This may seem like an instinctive thing to do as there is pain but by using your hands you are actually beginning a process of self-healing. And from here a magical set of things are set in motion: warmth to soothe and reduce pain; a signal also goes to increase endorphins; more blood flow to carry away the bruised blood cells and relieve the stress on skin tissues, and many other things to speed up the mending process. It really does do this. The problem is we never keep our hands on the area long enough for this healing process to really kick in and achieve its maximum benefit. We hold our hands there for a bit, until the initial pain starts to subside, we give a last little rub and move on. There is always something else we need to do in our busy lives. But please, next time give this a try. Keep your hand or hands on the area for longer and it will definitely help with the healing process.

Step Two is all about developing a greater connection to your body and in doing so you begin to gain a greater understanding of the language of your body and how it communicates. And once you have this communication you can actively work on healing different areas that you may have been previously unaware of. If you practise this step daily you will find that the tingling or other sensations restart pretty quickly for whatever part of your body you are focusing on. If you then allow this to travel anywhere, you can pay attention to the areas it moves to. For example, if you feel something in your shoulder, whether it be tingling or heat or an ache, keep your attention on this part. You might find that it becomes painful and that the pain increases the more you focus on it. Please try and stick with it and allow the pain to build. It is actually going through different processes and healing itself.

This is your body's way of communicating and now you are able to actively respond and build a rapport. With this increased awareness you can begin to help and heal many problems and issues. So just keep practising for a few days and you should notice many little improvements not only in your body but the mind will seem better too. It only takes a few seconds to do this and at some point, it *will* become automatic for you.

*****

Physical pain

Usually, physical pain requires our immediate attention – it is something that shouldn't be ignored but in reality, often is (depending on the severity, of course). We have become very good at ignoring the warning signs, often learning to live with the pain or pushing it aside. These are things that could develop later on in life and become much worse if left untreated. Yet this is just another example of how our busy lifestyles and busy minds do us no favours at all.

We can all be guilty of leaving things, especially when it comes to ourselves. Putting yourself first does not come easy. We have the mindset that 'I can manage' or 'I can cope' and that looking after yourself is in some way selfish! Being Omni will quietly help you address this and by healing yourself first, those around you will also greatly benefit. By building a rapport with your body, you will find that instead of living with something, you can do something to change it.

> *"We are the best at helping others if we look after our own needs first. This is where Omni has played a big part for me. The simplicity of the steps, especially the breathing one, have been easy for me to adopt at any given moment. Unlike mediation and some of the other lengthy relaxation processes, I find I can tap into Being Omni and go about my day. It reminds me that self-care is not selfish. You cannot pour from an empty cup. Taking care of yourself is vital."*
>
> *Louise Adams*

Say you have an ache in your back. Begin to put your thoughts and attention on the area where you can feel the most pain or discomfort. Hold your attention here. One of the most common things to happen is that the pain intensifies, but please persevere. It really is helping your body via its own healing methods, with no side effects whatsoever. The pain may get worse but stick at sensing it. It may well shoot or move to another area – follow it and sense again. You might get the same effects: pain increases and then moves. Keep following it and it will end up at the original site of the problem. As you are tracking the pain through your body, each area is being healed and cleared. Once you have found the source or original site, then this is when the most effective healing can take place.

Journal opportunity ~ Make a note of anything you experience while practising this step and whether it begins to help or change things in any way.

*****

Emotional and mental hurts

More often than not, many of our problems, pains or discomforts stem from a more indirect source. And that source is emotional hurts or scars which can manifest physically. The way we think does affect the body. It is the same when we feel an emotion.

Up until this point in our lives, most of us have lived in our heads, where thoughts alter how we feel emotionally doing our bodies no favours at all. The media and society where we live also have a big part to play in our emotional and mental responses. Many of our thoughts are media-driven in the sense it dictates or influences current trends, obsessions and fashions: what to eat, what to drink, what's healthy, what isn't, what you should wear, how your body should look and so on. It endlessly impacts our thinking, decisions and emotional states.

Worse still is the fact that news travels to us from around the world in seconds, which can affect us emotionally, changing our mood which in turn impacts our body dramatically. Our emotional reactions to films or TV programmes, whether good or bad, affect the body.

If you consider how many emotional reactions you can have throughout the day, it can be a bit of a rollercoaster. Every emotional reaction you have will have an effect. One of the best books to help with how we react to things is *The Four Agreements* by Don Miguel Ruiz. It explains how four agreements can dramatically improve different aspects of our lives and how we react to things. And for us in the Omni world, we use the four agreements firstly on our self: 'I will not take things personally' rather than 'Don't take things personally'.

Stress, depression, fears and anxieties are now commonplace in every one's life to some degree or other. Stress makes us feel sick to the stomach. Anxiety impacts the head and heart so it affects our nervous system and sets off our endocrine system which goes to work trying to rebalance. Yet because we are still attached to our primal and primate ways of being, adrenaline floods our systems meaning we should fight or take flight. But in our modern-day world we do neither, we just worry more and more. Our bodies can only take so much.

When you are practising Step Two, you may have some sort of flash back to an incident in your past, and you begin to see an image of an event in your mind's eye. It could be something that happened, an accident, or even someone saying something you were hurt by. This is the health problem's start point, and once you have seen this, it no longer holds any power over you or your body and the problem is fixed once and for all.

When you begin to know yourself, you also elevate and evolve out of the parts attached to our primal and primate systems of the pecking order and then you become steadier emotionally and more okay with being yourself.

*****

Energy Blocks

When something happens that emotionally affects us, the reaction surges through our bodies and into our energy fields and leaves a scar. If you have a CD with a scratch on it, distorted playback happens and you soon get rid of it. But with us, the emotional scars we have are often repeated (through memory triggers) and the scratch deepens and becomes a block to a happy life. As you practise Being Omni, this is greatly reduced and will even disappear.

> *"Free from the mind's interference, Being Omni allows my body's natural healing mechanisms to function at their best and I believe this can begin a healing process*

for any ailment - physical, mental, or spiritual. And if something cannot be healed then Being Omni allows for a deep acceptance of this and helps light a path forwards to turn this to our advantage. For me personally, Being Omni has helped me overcome some difficult emotional baggage where my teacher, Robert Light, has helped me discover certain tools to bring about an Omni state to overcome these challenges, whether it be singing, toning, breathing, sensing the body within, certain personal mantras and so on and I am continuously grateful for this help and support. I feel I am much more myself day-to-day and much more comfortable being me – happy, healthy and becoming more and more free of the interference of the mind. It's an ongoing journey, of course, but for me, Being Omni is very much a part this and will continue to help me learn, grow, heal and truly live each day, shining my light in the world."

Thoby Davis

*****

Benefits to Step Two

Making this step part of your daily routine means you will continually learn from it and it really will help with the way you live and experience your life.

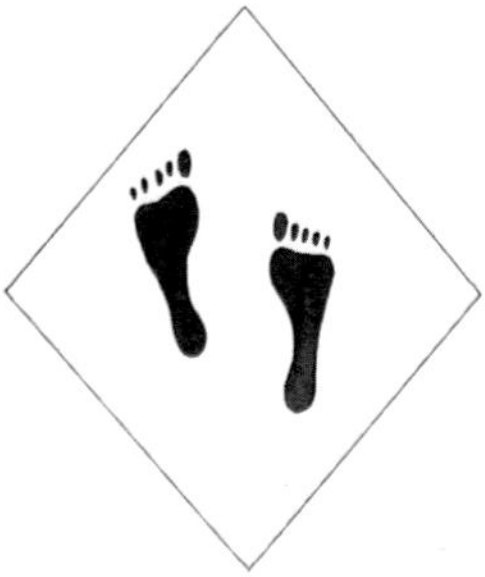

It's all about...

- o waking up the nervous system.
- o reconnecting to your body.
- o activating your energy system by bringing it into the body.
- o accessing and living more and more in the reality of your moments.
- o reducing the mind's influence and mind-created issues by a pre-occupied mind. You use the mind to focus on breathing and sensing.
- o learning the difference between mind based (conditioned) responses and actual real time body responses = accessing your truths.
- o learning a new language ~ the language of the body.
- o decreasing your mind space which simultaneously enables your central nervous system to function better with energy flowing from head to feet in consecutive bursts.

And when your central nervous system functions better, this also benefits many systems within your body. Alongside this, because the mind's harmful thinking is reduced pro rata, you will experience feeling a lot more relaxed which, in turn, helps your body heal.

∞

Understanding Energy

As we are beginning to experience the true relationship between body and mind, it would also be useful to explore how the energy part comes into play as it is a crucial part of the picture. We can better understand this energy part and perhaps why it has taken a back seat, when we look at the earliest stages of our existence.

*****

How I came to be and what I am

During conception, where a sperm travels to meet an egg (although there is nothing really great in this activity - it happens a lot and is pretty hit and miss), sometimes cosmic conditions are just right and as the egg and sperm meet, a flash or spark explodes within the egg and at the same time a life begins. Three things make one: two earthly, one cosmic.

A form begins made from squishy earth materials which keep multiplying, morphing and transforming. Depending on a few things, it keeps morphing until the spark makes contact with its host spark and then a form becomes fixed and a being begins, me as it happens.

I become more and more solid; all sorts of materials gather - water, air, liquids and matter. I grow and grow and then I am born. At this point I have moved from a liquid breather to an air breather and instead of being in the safety of a warm, dark place, I am thrust into the light.

As with our DNA, which has many things attached within it like the history of our origin, there are other things that are 'set' within us. Because I was born in a certain place, I will have an imprint of its magnetic energies. These line up with my central nervous system and the ghost meridian system. The date and time of birth also leave a mark in my energy fields. Then they give me a name which similarly has things attached to it. Think of the process of naming or creating an identity - what expectations or attachments the parents might have and the reasons they pick a particular name. Gosh, it's tedious! Why can't I just be me?

A human being relies upon the elements for its survival: air, water, food (fuel), fire which is how the human body functions. We breathe, we eat (earth things), we drink, the stomach produces heat to consume some of the food, and we have natural waste system where things should go back into the earth, not the sea!

I have a real, solid physical body made up of the above. And somewhere within, we have that spark that caused all this to happen. This is like a nuclear plant inside us producing the energy of life. We have a nervous system which is real and tangible and running in tandem with it is the energy system. It is subtly connected with our nervous system and mediates with the spark.

Up to a certain age, the mind is not too conditioned and has a fair amount of free range and play to enjoy learning and developing – this is a creating stage. But more rules and regulations happen and begin to impinge on us. From the age of about three onwards, the mind begins to separate from the connections to the spark and we move slowly from our bodies into our minds. Sadly, at some point, we sever this connection and become purely mind-orientated.

Therefore, a human being is far, far more than just a physical form. There is a complete double energy system within that has unlimited power and it is something we can all re-connect to.

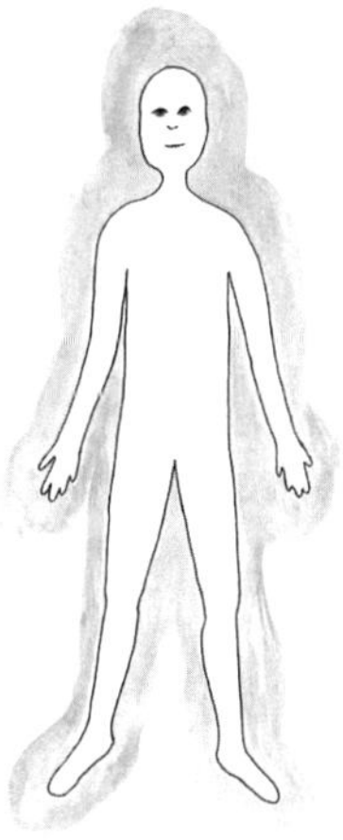

*****

Our need to define and label

It's also important at this point to look at our need to define and label. Here we are explaining the energy part and this is useful, but to become a whole being, it helps to not see each part of us as separate things.

If we imagine that once something is defined and labelled, the mind then allots a box to it. It's defined but is in a box and has therefore become separate. Everything is neat and tidy...but boxed in. It is exactly the same with a human being. We keep dividing it up into many parts and systems: mind and body, spirit and soul, higher self and energy part and so many more labels to define this or that. And in doing so, by separating everything, we move further and further away from our own true self.

By practising Being Omni, we live more and more in our moments and the need to define and label reduces proportionally because we are *doing* more rather than *thinking* of doing. If you sense your feet and note how they feel, it is doing rather than thinking of doing that forms a greater mind-body connection. Your feet become more of an active part rather than a separate part.

The body can take care of itself once you begin to care for it and nurture it. Our bodies are wonderful things. They are very complex in how they function and the less pressure they have from the mind means our bodies are much improved; they last longer and your health should get better and better.

*****

Your Energy System

Our five senses are our external, physical contact points. The central nervous system receives this sensory information and basically controls the body's response. This nervous system runs on minute electrical impulses that go right through our bodies, and certain nerve plexus points (which are a bit like roundabouts on roads) are where several nerve lines join up which allows, for example, our sense of touch to work. Your energy system is running parallel to this and is not necessarily connected physically. This energy system floats about within our bodies.

◊ *Energy is an amorphous mass – it doesn't take form or shape but fits within the body.*

We know a lot about the human body and we know a fair bit about the mind, but not really much about the energy system that the body actually has.

To help with our understanding of this, if you can envisage how broadband works it will give us a huge clue. Originally, the old telephone wire system had six wires but only used three or four of them. Now the signal that was going through the wire also created another set of signals outside of the cable. Every single wire has three to four waves of flowing electricity around it, a bit like magnetic fields hovering above and flowing around the wire. All the electric wires in your house have magnetic fields pulsing around them (some of which are harmful). It is these signals from the telephone wire that we now use for broadband.

The six wire (6x6) has thirty-six connections hence most homes have a good broadband connection. If we relate this to your body, each nerve line also has waves or pulses of energy around them. Some call these meridian flows, where each nerve line connects to a plexus point and it splits off and goes in different directions. In meridian flow, a nodal point is when an acupuncturist places a needle along these lines and they either short out the flow or increase it. It's the same with acupressure treatments. Many healing systems and healers trace or sense these lines to find and clear blocks, helping the body to restore health.

If we look at when you are in the womb, we can see that with the development of a baby's early consciousness, it is also reacting to or experiencing an energy interchange. After a set time, your early consciousness begins to form and it responds to your mother's moods (her highs and lows). You are not thinking here but starting off your feeling and sensing way of being.

If the mother is happy, energy-wise it feels lighter and good to the baby. If things go wrong for the mother, she becomes heavy and down and so your world darkens and becomes heavier. Even though you do not understand your mother's processes, you do begin to have a sense of energy interchanges. These basic energy exchanges can be felt and experienced on a physical, sensory level where the body feels lighter or heavier. We can explore this in relation to your immediate physical world too. For example, if you are feeling sad or down, your body will actually be heavier on the chair.

If we look at this in relation to the mind, we can see how the mind, which is the energy of the brain, can affect the body. When something happens, we react – good or bad – and it is these reactions, the highs and lows, which leave traces all through the body and in the body's surrounding energy fields. It is to this we should look for some of the causes of our illnesses. For example: anger, resentment or annoyance, all seem to affect our livers. Emotional hurts tend to linger in the stomach area, whereas lack of self-confidence or self-worth affects the upper chest and so on.

Practising Step Two, sensing and feeling, will help you with self-healing and clearing away some of the traces that cause physical problems. Your body's energy system is part of it – each cannot be separate as they are all intrinsically connected and make the whole. You will find that your senses are heightened, they are tuned up so to speak. And as your ability to tune into these flows and signals increases, your sense of internal and external energies begins to function better.

◊ *If only we truly knew our true self then most illness, dis-ease would not happen.*

We will explore these inner-outer sensing abilities in more detail as we move into Step Three and look at how our internal and external worlds are connected.

As above, so below

As within, so without

It's good to know that Step Three starts to happen automatically as you practise the first two steps. This happens because we are becoming more awake to ourselves and then our links and connections with the world around us increase. For the most part, because we have come to live solely from our mind and a thinking perspective, our interactions with the world around us are also a mind-orientated one. This very similar to how the body and mind have become detached, as explained in the previous step. By perceiving the world from the mind's point of view, a separateness between the internal (you) and the external (world) occurs.

We like to think we're connected because, after all, it's our immediate reality – it's the world in which we live. In truth, rarely do we experience a real interaction or engagement with the world, where a rapport is established and communication is a two-way thing. Step Three changes this so we can discover how to experience our reality in a completely different way, where we stop being just observers, stamping our big, heavy footprints everywhere and simply admiring beautiful views, and instead actually participate in and communicate with this world.

When we practise Step Three, we are attuning our five senses and begin to use them differently to before. This blurs the separateness and the gap between the external and internal reduces so they begin to act as one. A dialogue is established ~ a language without words ~ and we live more harmoniously and synchronised with the world around us.

Our energy part also begins to participate in our daily lives. We are much, much more than just our physical bodies and there are parts of us which are not limited to this. We have an energy part and also an inbuilt sonar system. We have thought tendrils and an electro-magnetic field to name just a few. And some of these can travel a very long way from our bodies.

With this step, we work with our ability to extend our energy part via a thought to connect to and get a 'sense of' a place or situation. This is a new way to use our thoughts as they are being consciously created and directed within that moment. The 'sense of' information is relayed back to us via the body and we can start to learn how to listen to the body's responses. The body is 100% reliable here. It has no fixed agendas. The body does not use words neither does it have logic within it. It does not know right from wrong so is not biased. It exists only in real time not mind time.

To have access to something completely reliable is pretty amazing, don't you think? To be able to tune into something that can never lie or deceive you is something I'm sure many of us have wished for. It's like having your own alethiometer[5] ~ in this way, your body becomes your very own truth-teller.

When we enter our own world of an energy being, it defies logic and reason and, because of this, it is very hard to write about and explain. As a species, humans have learnt to need and expect rational and logical answers to things. For the moment, try and suspend the need for logic and reason and just go with the flow. An open mind is needed here, and please remember, it is about the *doing rather than the thinking.*

[5] An alethiometer is a fictional object from Phillip Pullman's 'His Dark Materials' trilogy. It allows certain people to know the answer to any question. The name comes from ancient Greek (alethia meaning truth and meter meaning measure).

Step Three

Sense of

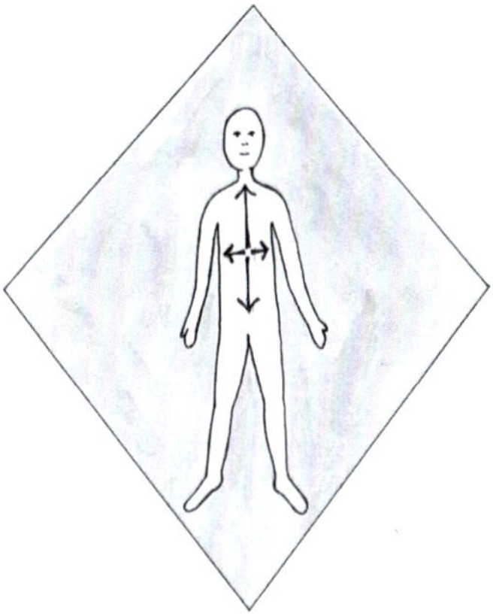

We can start to practise this step with the following question...

'How does this room feel right now?'

The wording is critical here – it signifies a specific place and time for you to work with.

When this question is asked, usually you will give a mind-based response very similar to that in Step Two. You might sit there for a while and get absolutely nothing or think, 'It feels fine to me'. But please, persevere.

It will help to break the area down further. Go back to the question, state it again in your mind or aloud and let's look at the room in sections.

For example, if you are sitting in your living room, split the room into an imaginary half, and then split it in half again so you end up with four quarters. Next, look at the first section and check which parts you can see clearly. You might find as you look at the other sections that even though you can see everything, some things might be unclear or blurry. Here is a good time to incorporate Omni breathing whilst still looking. With practice, you will be able to see all parts of the room equally. When you can see each part clearly, use this question for each section: 'How does this section of the room feel?' and so on.

One of the main things affected will be your weight, where your body touches solid things like the chair or where your feet touch the floor. Our five senses work as early warning systems from the body not the mind. Depending on whether the energy of an area is fine or harmful to us in some way, your body will subtly lean in response to thoughts on how the room is. The five senses, when combined with the energy part, are like a radar wave that travels from your body and each then receives a signal. It sounds far-fetched but the more Omni you become, this will become more plausible.

Here, you are learning how to direct your thoughts and utilise your energy sensing capabilities beyond your physical body to receive a *sense of* the room that your Omni state can understand and respond to.

If you go back to the explanation about being able to sense the mother's mood when you are a baby, you can now actually apply this to your current external world and, as you learn to pay more attention to your body, you will get to sense the body's subtle movements and shifts in relation to your external world and internal thinking. Make a note of anything within your body you become aware of: a pull or a push on the body's alignment; different pressures (often occurring in parts of your head); a difference of body weight either heaviness or lightness; sets of subtle sounds; a pull or shift to the right or left or any other way your body reacts.

Each part of the room will also have a sound or vibration associated with it. As you are getting a sense of the room, you might be able to hear this. It's a bit like tinnitus where different tones or pitches start ringing in your ear.

At first, much of the information is incredibly subtle and because this ability has not been used for so long, it will take time to develop. It's a bit like fine tuning: you are tuning up your senses and this does not happen overnight. You have been absent or disconnected since birth with reference to this arena. But if you practise this step as often as you can, your insight and awareness of the different ways your body relays information, will definitely evolve.

This is a language that allows you to communicate properly with your body within the reality of your present flowing moments. And, you also begin to develop a more connected, balanced and beneficial relationship between your internal and external worlds.

*****

Listening to your body's responses

◊ *If you have practised Step Two, feeling and sensing, you will know that your body's reactions happen independently and honestly unlike your mind and heart ever will. This is because the body exists in real time and these are reactions from your present reality. Yes, some things are very hard to swallow or take on board, but nevertheless they are true. It is rare that we look within – but your body will always tell your truth.*

Many external factors impinge upon us and affect our bodies, for good or bad: electricity and Wi-Fi; what we eat and drink; the air that we breathe. Our interactions with others also have an impact be it emotionally or mentally. This happens because we have not yet moved out of our primal and primate instincts for survival and we live in a world where the alpha is still at the top. We like to think otherwise but nevertheless it is true. Being Omni will help you begin to have a level playing field and, as the two worlds merge, the impact of these external factors decreases.

By learning how your thoughts and energy sensing capabilities can pick up and tune in more adeptly to your external environment, you can then actively reduce the impact certain external factors have on you. For example, as you receive a sense of something or someone, you can then change it by clearing it, healing it or creating a shift. Even just re-connecting will be beneficial to you.

Now you've had a go at sensing your immediate environments, let's have a go with other external factors in your life.

For the moment, we will refer to four basic physical reactions and this is how we can usually interpret them:

Heavier = wrong
Lighter = right
Lean back = wrong
Lean forward = right

Ask the question, 'How does my home / house feel?' You could just think about where you live or use the words, 'Where I live'. It's good to experiment with different ways of phrasing things so you can find what works for you.

Firstly, does your body react?

Is it heavier? Lighter? Does it lean slightly forwards or move backwards?

Using this step for your home environment can help in many ways. It will certainly reduce the effects of such things as Wi-Fi and electricity.

You can practise this with all manner of different things. For example, the food you eat. If you pick up an item of food, your body will react. It might lean backwards or forwards slightly. It is up to you, of course, what you do with this information. We all eat and drink things that aren't always very good for us! However, by learning how your body responds to certain things, you could then clear them. This is just a directed thought or instruction, ‘Clear this food’ or ‘Clear this drink’ which improves how it is taken in by your body. You might also find that your body will communicate something it needs and you will *feel* like eating or drinking something or find that the image of a certain food keeps appearing in your mind.

As we progress with Being Omni, the wonderful thing is that a natural clearing begins to happen. Say, for example, the chef at your favourite restaurant is having a bad day, and you go there and order a meal. As it is being served, it gets cleared and actually, so does the chef. Not only is your food cleared but you have actually helped the chef too. It’s a win-win for all.

Next, try and get a sense of where you work.

> *“For me, when I thought of work, my body became quite heavy and sluggish. This might be an emotional or mental block. I might have been worrying about something or stressed because I hadn’t finished a certain task. Here, I immediately did Omni breathing and a bit of Step Two. When I thought of work again, my body was no longer heavy so I had cleared that problematic part of my thinking away.”*
>
> *Heather Light*

How about when you think of certain family members? One at a time, of course. Pay attention to how, with each thought, your body reacts.

Whatever information you get back, for example, if you think of someone close to you and you feel heavier, do the Omni steps and at the same time send them lightness or healing or wellness. It really helps to clear the problem for them or perhaps shift something that was between you in the relationship.

But please remember, the answers are for that moment in time, and only that time!

There are so many different ways to experiment with this step and the more you do, the more you will experience this new way of communicating, and the more you and all that surrounds you will benefit.

∞

The Magic (Genie) Within

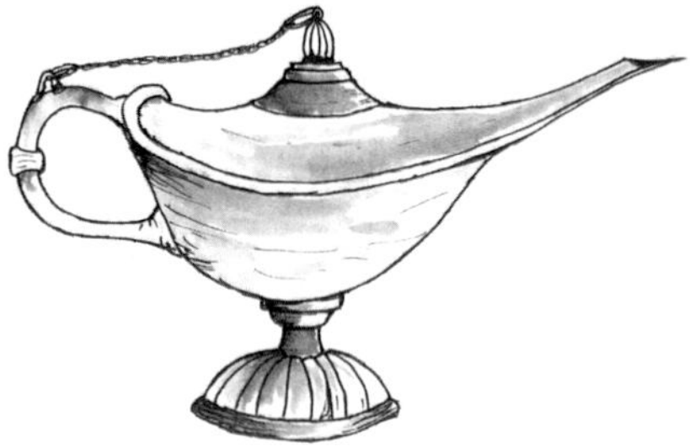

Does it have a use? I ask myself. And *yes*, is the answer. It's a life-saver in many ways. When you are present in time and space, your body is well and so are you.

As we begin to use our five senses in a Being Omni way, our internal senses also heighten. Hunches, gut instinct (being the two most basic), intuition and a deeper sense of knowing are such senses. These types of 'inner awareness' have sadly been lacking in humankind for generations but they are totally normal skills or abilities that everyone has.

Really, it is not as strange as it sounds. We actually use instinct and intuition all the time, we just don't always know what to do with the information.

We have a sense of others, situations and events, and this is inherent within us. It has just become a rather neglected and unused part of us. For example, you would have perhaps experienced that a certain person does not *feel* right, or you get a sense that a place is either right or wrong. You don't like it here or that area feels cold or gives you a chill or something begins to affect your mood and you're not sure why. Or even when you think of someone and soon after you actually bump into them or they call out of the blue. People have endless examples of these kinds of occurrences! Many will put it down to coincidence or just think that it's spooky or strange when actually it is a natural, inherent ability of how you are reacting to different things in your external environment.

By practising Step Three, our interaction with the external world increases but not in a pressured or forced way, it just happens. As we are no longer reacting the way the mind would want us to, we are gaining control in many areas.

◊ *This step really will help you to find your own answers and truths, allowing you access to the magic within.*

"Being Omni quietens my mind allowing a change in my perspective and leaving me a feeling of strength to work with from any point. The Omni steps are easy and the more they are practised, they become an automatic life choice. As with Omni breathing, one becomes fluid and in-line with one's day to day energy. The mind is not in charge so cannot decipher the changes that have happened. As the mind quietens and relaxes, it allows one's body to take over, bringing with it trust in the self

and strength in that trust. This leads to the very best of experiences even in the very worst circumstances. Omni gives me the opportunity to begin again over and over. To begin by experience and to acknowledge the power I can easily access – simply, methodically, limitlessly."

Tracy Davies

A person will already know before they go somewhere if it is safe for them but rarely do we listen to these feelings.

All my life I have been very lucky to have a sort of early warning system that I listen to. While I am with other people and they are talking away, I receive a noise in my right ear if they are speaking truly and if false, it is in my left ear. In most cases, it is infallible. At the same time, I can feel and sense their energy fields expanding or contracting, and often I can see a colour change in these fields around a person. At the same time, my body will either move backwards or forwards in response to their words. It may also lean slightly left or right in response to certain things. The other thing of note is it gets heavier or lighter in response to words too, so I have a few things that tell me if it is safe or not. Actually, once or twice my car just will not start, and even the AA man can't get it to work! This happens if I am planning on going somewhere and later on in the news I hear about a car crash on the route I would have taken. So early warning systems do really work and *everyone* has them.

People who know me or learn the things I teach, make excuses like I cannot see or feel like you do. I would not want anyone to see the things I do full stop - it is a gift and a curse at the same time. But every one of you can sense and feel things without a shadow of a doubt!

We are all part of the energy exchanges of Earth. Every single thing has an energy field we can sense. If 'x' is the start point of a tremor or earthquake, our energy fields can pick this up days before it actually occurs.

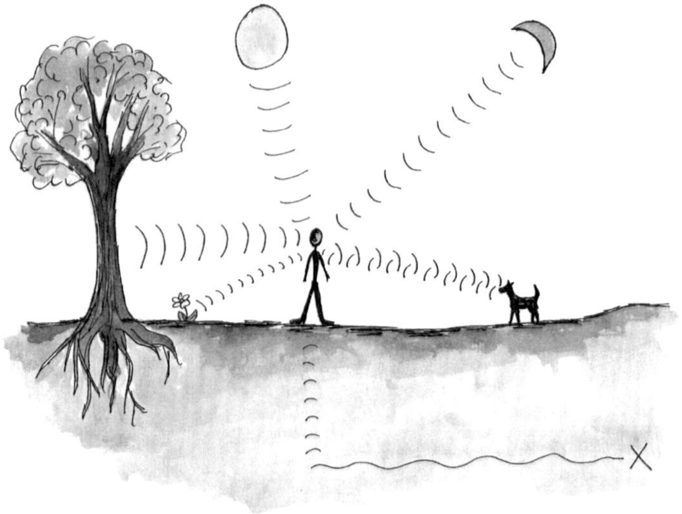

Omni's simple steps allows a natural return to these inner-outer abilities bit by bit as it should be. If you are Being Omni, then listen and feel the subtle changes your body is going through. If you are Being Omni, your body will be reacting to these words – does it lean forward or backward?

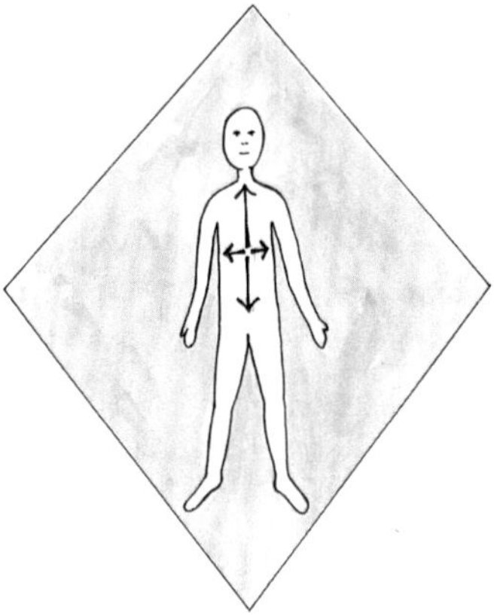

*****

Omni is the simplest of things, yet your Way forward is complex
because you have only your mind to begin this journey
But as you near steps 1 to 3 in Being Omni
Your mind and thoughts will have
Changed to living and being
And you are becoming as
oNe

*****

You will find that within each step there are many levels and, as you go through this book, you will revisit the steps in different ways. Each time you do this, it enhances your Omni state of being. And so begins your journey of self-awareness and an improved sense of self, where you begin to feel better and much more in control of your own life.

> *"The breathing step allows me to slow my mind down and regain control over its incessant chatter and worry. Slowly but surely my heart rate falls and it's as if a weight has been lifted from my chest as the anxieties melt away. Thinking is replaced with clarity of mind, and I enter a different state of being. My vision and hearing improve and, generally, I feel more myself. I take great pleasure in Step Two as I begin to feel my own energies and begin to come home to myself and feel more "me". With the third step, I feel as If I am engaging with and active within my world and the world around me. Everything seems more alive and interesting – my curiosity grows and my sense of wonder increases. For me, this is the best way I know to quickly and easily free myself from the egoic mind, to become present and whole and to be alive within my moments. Being Omni doesn't cost a penny, it takes very little "time" and the rewards are priceless. A whole being and sincere thank you to Robert Light and Heather Light for sharing with us these life-changing and life enhancing steps to Omni – being my true self, in my moments, alive and free."*
>
> *Bethan Williams*

∞

Why has nothing before worked before?

Personally, I have been giving talks and workshops for a long time. When I had finished the talk, everyone would go outside to say goodbye. The talk had gone really well where everyone was uplifted, bright and shiny. As people left, I would watch as they walked back to their cars and even as they were walking away, I could see the light grow dimmer within those wonderful people.

Why?

Immediately, thoughts of going home...having to cook dinner... thinking about the family who are waiting and, worse still, getting up early tomorrow to go to work or thinking the traffic home will be awful. As soon as these different thoughts kicked it, it switched the light firmly off. They were no longer living in the present flowing moments but by letting the mind take over with past and future thoughts meant nothing had changed!

> ◊ *The point of power and change is in your present moment, not tomorrow nor yesterday or whenever, but now. Your point of enlightenment is right now in your present moment.*
>
> *Louise Hay, Heal your Body*

Even when all the New Age thinking burst forth onto the everyday scene and became almost mainstream and prevalent for those people seeking advice, it did not really help them.

They would attend courses, talks, workshops, visit Gurus, read some of the thousands of books on self-help, all to attain wholeness, oneness and freedom. People paid a fortune to go to some talks by famous self-help Gurus, and yet ended up in the same place or state of mind afterwards. Sometimes, even though they had learnt so much and felt so much better with all the others, as they left the room the talk was held in, even before the door had closed, all that seemed to vanish. For others, the feeling better bit may last a day, a week or longer but the problems never really went away.

Always it was the mind and its way of thinking that destroyed the light within. I have never been happy with this so I kept working on the content of my talks and courses to ease this terrible mind burden and swapped and changed until I found a way that truly works and gives everyone the freedom of being themselves.

Omni is guaranteed to work every time.

- o What happens to you when I make that statement?
- o What are your thoughts?
- o More importantly how does your body react to those words?

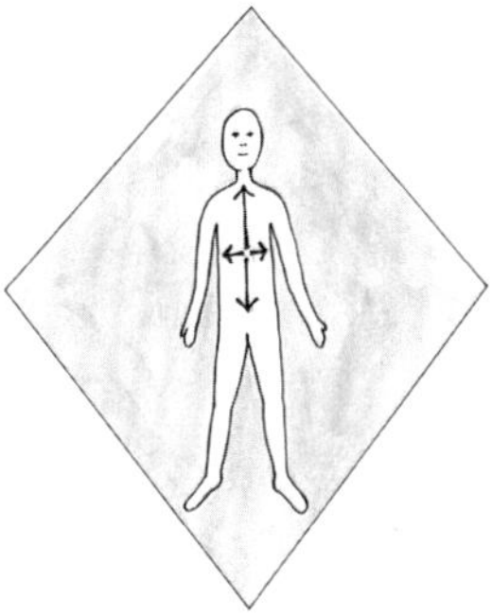

Why is the mind and how we think able to do this? How and why does it destroy the light within?

Remember your mind, thoughts and thinking have millions of agendas based upon your life so far. Your thoughts, coupled with emotion, confirm and strengthen these agendas. Your body, on the other hand, lives purely within your moments and does not have a single agenda.

Please be patient with my words and listen and feel and sense rather than judge or want to justify what you have been led to believe.

∞

The Mind

To explain why the body's information is so much better than the mind, we have to go right back in our history and look at how we have learnt to become so dependent and reliant on the mind and thinking...

When we were little, we used our imagination and visualisation a lot which came free and unbidden. Nothing was really fixed and our internal and external worlds were interchangeable. But as the reality of our world dawned on us, things changed and our interactions with our world began to affect us emotionally and leave scars within us (within the energy self). We used imagination less and less and instead memories started to form. These are either good or bad, but each one is placed in the mind as a reference point.

Each of these reference points then become fixed points on our timelines and in doing so, a fixed set of reactions is formed. This is how allotted time slots begin. Once something becomes allotted to a specific time slot, we consciously or unconsciously (knowingly or unknowingly) refer back to it and it informs or directs or dictates how we respond in the present.

The image below represents a very basic time line where every dash signifies an event or occurrence. If you created your own, you would have many more dashes. Some events, of course, are more significant than others but the point is, a dash (time slot) is created for every single thing that impacts you or you have an emotional reaction to. You can perhaps now visualise how many dashes one person alone would need!

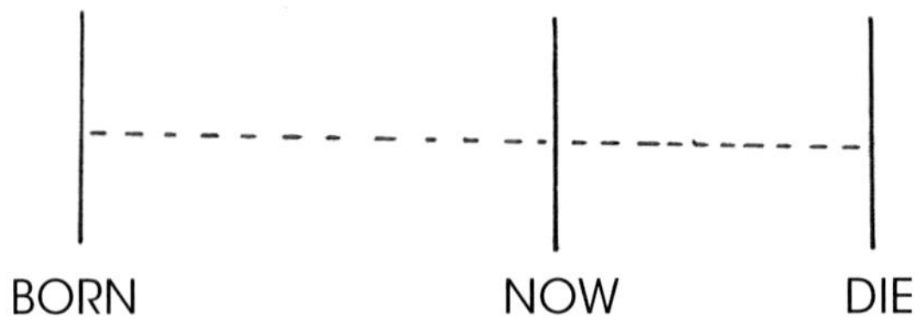

Therefore, the mind holds or stores everything that has ever happened to you. And this is how it can influence your current thinking and being and living. It also incorporates all the future events that you have conceived (the time slots between NOW and DIE). Everything you do, everything that happens to you, the mind quickly runs through every conceivable scenario based upon the information from these time slots and calculates what is best for you to keep you safe. Consequently, this has the majority impact determining how you act or respond.

The mind has some pretty strong agendas with our hearts and emotional counterparts faring no better. It's doing its best but the mind's programs are slightly wrong and very out of date.

It is because we live and react from *known* perspectives that it causes us to stay locked in old ways of being and reacting. This is why it's often so difficult for us to change as we have fixed habits and mindsets.

Omni is quite a shock for the mind because it believes that answers or how to react, have to be evaluated from past experience to find safe solutions in the now. This never really allows you to experience things from an open mind to something new. Yes, you can book a holiday to new place and a new experience will happen but you will always experience it from your mind's eye view. We could write a whole book on this but it is not really necessary – our need to know or define things really does hold us back from growing.

As you continue to use Being Omni, the need to know diminishes and changes into experiences that we have and, whether they are good or bad, they are no longer stored as memories but as happenings. You will still have good recall, (probably a better one at that!) and also greater emotional stability. And by living more in your present moments, it actively reduces the amount of mind related referrals from your time line so they no longer influence your present decisions or reactions. You approach each situation with a clean, new perspective: we react more than think of reacting. And when your mind begins to live in the same time and space as your body, you will have arrived home.

There's still much to do and to grow even more ~ this is just the beginning!

*****

Words and Mindsets

Our thoughts and how we think are inextricably linked with the words we use and these words quickly become mindsets. Mindsets are when our thoughts travel along known and fixed paths. Without even realising, we are conditioned and programmed into thinking, feeling and knowing in set ways and patterns.

We have a name for everything we know. Name or word = a thought and thinking of. Then words become inexhaustibly capable of inflicting or remedying. Words and what they mean to each of us, can cause great harm or joy within anybody.

One of the Being Omni exercises is shifting and sifting past, present and future into awareness of and living in the nows and moments. The mind and thinking, uses and mixes past into present to evaluate what you need to do to keep yourself safe. So, your past has enormous influence on your present.

What was, really does not have any bearing on what is.

A child's mind is always discovering new things. However, most after the age of nine today, have lost this. My wife has always said I am like a child - a parcel arrives and I am excited to open it (even if it isn't my parcel!). In company, I am drawn to children as they like to play, explore or discover new things; they always have new ways of doing and playing. Some parents rediscover this when their babies become toddlers and infants and learn to play once more. But this is soon lost in the seriousness of life and sadly both parents and children grow up too quickly.

Also, the words children learn from their parents become their way of life forever. We believe what we are told. Some children do question but it is pointed out by the adults not to do this. A child's question 'Why?' should never be ignored or put off till later. But we all end up with, 'This is the way it is' and we sort of build up an image or accept this is the norm.

Words are wonderful things, of course. It's what they mean to each of us and how the mind evaluates the words and puts them into context that determines how we feel. But can you look at things and not label what you see?

*****

The mindset with cancer

When told they have cancer, a person has a mindset that it leads to death. The consultant also has a set of thoughts that this outcome will happen. Yet a hope may spring forth - you can have an operation to remove the cancer - we will cut it out. Yet it might have already spread, so we will give you chemotherapy and radiotherapy to eradicate what has spread. This works for some cancers and some people live a long time afterwards plus there is always a new expensive drug you can take to help. Alongside all the conventional treatments, a new way of reducing set mind patterns is much needed. Unfortunately, as the mind prefers negative ways of thinking based upon what it knows, the mindsets of the patient and of other people still go on and, for some, death becomes the only option.

Yet what causes cancer? What is the very first step in it starting?

Diet? Smoking? Where you live or work? External energies? There are many, many reasons why cancer starts and one may also be about how you think and feel. Certain events leave a scar on us - a deep etching right through the physical into the very core within us and the poison begins.

Your words have become your truths – they define the way you live your life and, in a way (a word), it defines you too!

By Being Omni, we begin to alter these mindsets which reduces the power of the words we use to create problems. No one consciously uses words to create these but somewhere the words create the thoughts and then the mind brings things into our reality.

> *"I have done well over the years taking part in yoga classes and reading mindfulness books. However, it was only when I started practising the Omni steps that I have found myself able to take an extra leap into wellness and feeling calm as my usual state of being. I have found that I have been able to easily change mindsets and habits in the last year. I feel incredibly grateful to have found a practice that has changed my life for the better in so many ways."*

Jenny Stone

*****

Thoughts and thinking

In early human types, there was not much in the way of thoughts or thinking; the primate and primal survival instincts were there before thought. Food number one, water number two, mate number three, shelter number four and so on. When all the food within a mile radius had gone, guess what? You had to move to another location. The alpha male nearly always formed a group because, after all, they would do whatever he said. An alpha is nearly always lazy and clever. Nothing different today – politicians and others in power decide what you do and when you do it. You go around thinking you have free will or free choice but no my friend, delusions run deep! So, in a way, the alphas were the first to start thinking. After thinking came planning and control, and as the groups got bigger, the alpha needed a deputy or two and so the human hierarchy or pyramid of power developed and is still used today.

Types of thoughts

Throughout any day, a person can have thousands of thoughts, some even have millions. The range of a person's thoughts is vast and, in most cases, very diverse. There is often no rhyme or reason to them: some are inspirational, others mundane and ordinary. But we have all learnt to think in logical, typically linear and direct ways. This happens because we experience one track results and ways of living. For example, when we are first born, we cry and either get fed or not, but we work out the best system and stick with it. One track = results.

Most of our thinking is based upon this first set but this leads us to think in tracks or ruts. How many times have you heard people say, 'I am stuck in a rut'? And the ruts we create and live in can be pretty hard to get out of. The increase in mental health issues and problems that no tablets or counselling will fix is testament to this. These are harsh but true statements. If you have ever taken any anti-depressants or even had counselling – did any of these really work?

Omni can and will.

Other types of thoughts are about things to do and things we have done. Occasionally, a random thought does pop into your mind – 'I will go and visit Amy today' – never realising that Amy had just thought about you! And even more seldom, a new, unbidden thought comes to mind. These are absolute gems but mainly we are too busy to engage with these, or we justify not listening to them.

Many of our thoughts are worries. How often do you worry, fret or stress about someone? Worrying about family happens in the mind; it is part of your thinking and thoughts. But the majority of our thoughts are about the everyday things. Let's take the average food shopping experience to look at this more closely.

It begins with a thought – 'I have to go food shopping.'

From this thought, other actions and thoughts occur. You may make a list, think about what meals to plan for, or whether you need any household items, snacks – it's nice to have some treats, oh yes, need to buy some flowers for so and so...hmmm... what time shall I go? When is the best time to go? And so on...

Now, supermarkets use psychology very effectively to make you buy extras. They move stuff around so you have to search for the things on your list, and in the process, you buy other things that you really don't need or want, but you have been made to buy them. Really there is no thinking done here, you just do what you are told. Yes, this is not nice to hear but that is how life is for many today. One day you will wake up.

Next time, try and stick to your list only. You only have to look at how much we consume and want more and buy more so inevitably we waste more. This is the culture of today and it has become our way of thinking and being.

Cookers, fridges, washing machines and all the other household appliances used to last a long time – now, some have designed a fatigue on breakdown parts so you always need to buy a new item. It's the same with TVs, iPads, phones, consoles, computers and laptops which are all constantly being updated. There are many ways we are convinced and cajoled into buying new updated versions; they are promoted as better and faster, and that is what we want. We want the best version so we keep buying and throwing things away. This is the never-ending consumer cycle which is keeping your attention on wanting and needing more.

The simple task of going shopping and the different thought processes around it, can reveal a great deal about the mind and about how we think and how we are conditioned.

A thought is either creative or destructive.

Sometimes a thought becomes manifest and does create the reality of the world you live within. When thoughts are backed with an emotional response they then exist within your mind as a memory. And this determines decisions you make now.

Since you were born, how many thoughts have your created? And what happens to those thoughts? Do they just disappear, fade away or dissolve? Are thoughts contained within your head? Or is there more to them that we are only beginning to realise? Do they reach further? Even to the thing you are thinking about?

If you are like me and are sceptical, try this experiment. Have a think about the people you may not have seen for a while and make a list of about ten of them. Have a look at this list once a day for a week and see if there is some form of contact with someone on that list.

Journal entry ~ Because of the way we think or have learnt to think, negative thinking is easier and far more powerful than positive thinking. Lots will disagree with this, so keep a thought journal for a few days, even a week. You don't need to write much, just mark a tick for positive thoughts and a cross for negative ones.

A good example of how we can see that negative thinking has more power is when we drive. If you use a car, for example, to go to work or to do a school run, then you will have sets of thoughts (much like the food shopping example). These sets of thoughts are your mindsets. You will think about whether you are late or even early. You will think about the traffic and the roads being busier at different times. Thoughts like, 'Oh it's going to be hard to park' or 'There will be congestion and road works after this'. And sure enough, it is busy, you do struggle to park and it is stressful. Just have a think about your internal dialogue and whether this is true for you.

Real-life experience will always give you a way to determine whether this is right and demonstrate to you the result of this way of thinking and being. Try it out by using a different set of thoughts. Change the way you think about the journey or the supermarket food shop by simply stating beforehand, 'I will have a good journey' or 'I will arrive on time'.

The next exercises are something I have been asking people to practise for many years.

Whilst teaching self and energy awareness, I would ask people to go to their usual supermarket at the busiest time, when they usually struggle to get parking space and have a go at changing their mindsets about it. By changing their inner dialogue or way of thinking, there was a 7/10 success rate. They found a parking space easily and the shopping experience was quick and stress-free - so this proved it did work in most cases. The ones that it did not work for had allowed an afterthought to sneak in! 'Oh, it's always too busy' or 'This won't work for me'. It is the same with if you drive a route with sets of traffic lights and ask that they are all green when you get there. This works too. Some will say, if everyone does this, there will be chaos, or cause others problems, but I can assure you, all travel becomes a lot smoother.

When we think of finding a parking space, something amazing actually happens. A part of your consciousness goes forward in time to create that space. You are at home visualising the parking space at a specific time, and when you get there, someone drives out of that space at the right time. In a way, you are manipulating a future event: you are adjusting time and space in the future. If you take away the thinking, step out of your old self and its conditioning, everyone can win.

Do a body check now – do you lean forwards or backwards?

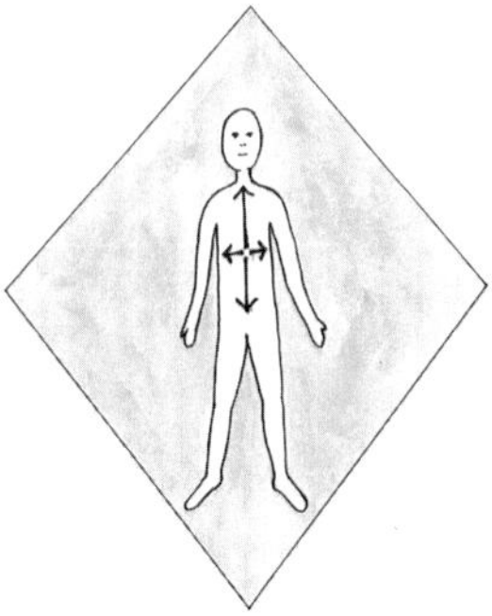

The impossible is always possible.

There are many examples of how and what you think determines the outcome – and hopefully you will experiment with this so you may have clearer evidence and actual experience of it.

The reason negative thoughts or what we try and avoid, have more power over the outcome than the positive ones is because we polarise our thinking. We are taught or trained by everything around us to try and be good and do the right thing.

I'm sure you would agree that in most cases we are taught to be good, to behave and to act in a way that is agreeable to others. This pushes us over to one side of ourselves. Say, for example, trying to be good equates to about 10–15% of this energy or power. The more you move towards only being good, the being bad side will grow or increase to meet the ratio (85%) and we actually give more emotional power to the things we dislike or hate or want to avoid. It is the most casual of thoughts that touch that part of us and consequently will have that 85% of power behind it. This means the mind is able to bring about the things you are trying so hard to avoid!

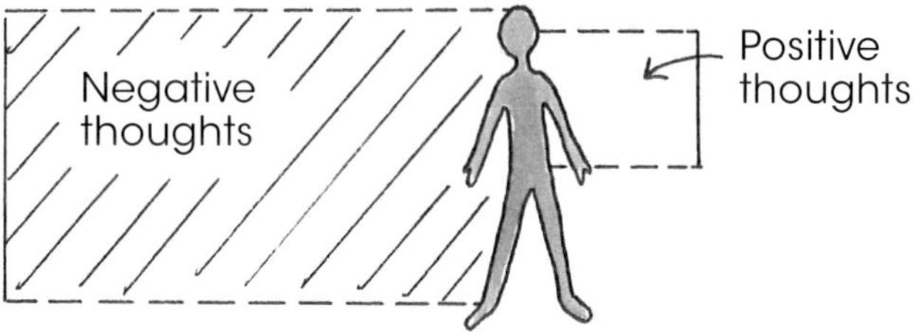

The idea of always trying to have a positive mental attitude seems a good idea but it if you invest all your energy into being positive, it is exactly the same as you trying to avoid being negative. It only divides you further and so becomes destructive and cannot be maintained by anybody. Full stop.

This is the first part of our training, our domestication. This is basically a system of agreements to encourage conformity. We enter into these agreements, with seemingly little choice here as wherever we look they are reflected and supported in every aspect of the world around us. As we take these on board our training into self-domestication[6] begins, and this is for life. The sets of opposites are then set in opposition: we separate them to such an extent that they become a dichotomy. Therefore, we live and grow up in a world of equals and opposites, and very much in the vein of complete duality.

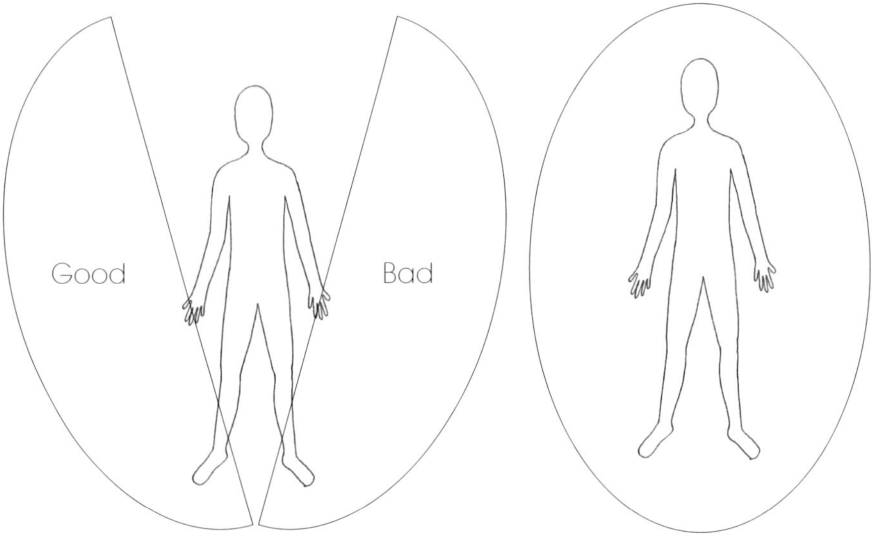

∞

[6] In the first part of 'The Four Agreements', Ruiz explains this process in detail. Re-read it a few times and try and get a sense of your self-domestication.

Duality

It is not necessarily the existence of opposites which causes problems but how we have interpreted and manipulated them. To understand why and how we have created this duality, we need to go back to the very beginning of our creation and even the creation of the universe itself.

When a person is conceived and the sperm penetrates the egg, creation begins with both the spark of light and the internal darkness, not too dissimilar to the big bang which began our present-day universe.

With the big bang and the start of evolution, the light went one way encompassing all that it found and the dark quietly moved in the opposite direction yet it too was all consuming. Light and dark began their journey; complete opposites but born out of the same substances.

Here we have the beginning of opposites, which for humans becomes the start of duality within. This happens because we set them up in opposition and live or experience our lives accordingly: good versus bad or love against hate; happy as preferable to sad and many more things like this.

And for each of us, as we go through life, every one of these opposites will have different levels and depths of meaning, confirming and augmenting the duality within.

*****

Love and Hate

Hate and love are words humans have created to fit our needs and to explain and justify if something is right or wrong.

Love is the simplest of things, and is very beneficial to you, yet each of us has our own complete view of love and what it is. Consequently, if you to seek to define love or use the word love, it always comes with connotations. To write about love or even have a discourse upon it, will never go far.

In Paulo Coelho's book, *The Pilgrimage*, one of the main characters explains the different types of love we experience and have developed. He does this to elucidate the problems and heartaches that are caused by people having a specific view on love. Each of us will experience different variations of love; it is not a straightforward emotion or feeling. We have unconditional love, a child's love of their parent, love of your partner, friendship, love of nature, animals – there are many, many different types of love. But if I asked you to love yourself, many would find it hard or difficult to do so, simply because you do not yet know yourself nor have you found yourself.

A baby just born, does not know love of its parent - it has to grow or be earned. It is a very contentious thing to write as the need to be loved is paramount in many. So, if you use the word love, we can see that it always comes with connotations. And in the world of opposites, if you have love then you will also have hate. As with the different types of love, there are also different depths of hate. Like day and night, they cannot be separated in our current contexts.

Love like Omni cannot be defined or contained within words. It is a rapport with the self or your external environment that happens in a moment and goes in a moment. But like most things, we want to own it or cling onto it. We begin to define or label and put a word to it. It then no longer functions properly but instead functions as a set of thoughts that trigger emotions and then sets of responses. Love in this context binds and controls us.

◊ *Less love = more love*

When you embark upon the Omni journey, these contexts are no longer needed. Omni and newness go hand in hand. It's not that you won't feel love, but you will experience it more and more in its truest form...within the flowing moments.

◊ *When we can learn to entwine love and hate then we begin and duality declines.*

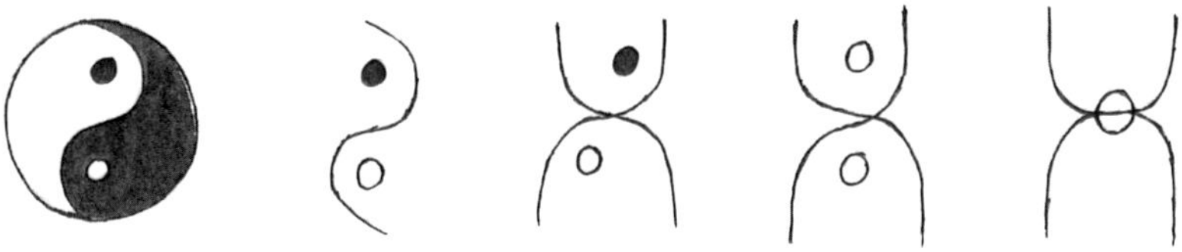

Far too long have we sought the light and ignored the dark yet both are present in our daily lives. Like the sun and moon that dance as one, although they both have different kinds of light both are perfectly matched to the earth's seasons and cycles.

As we grow up, we are told to be good and push away anger and bad thoughts which at the very beginning of our lives are as close as peas in a pod. Those around us and who we look to for guidance, as they do not know any better as yet, also force this apart within us.

However, every single human being has the capacity to be good or bad. We only have to watch the news to see this. The great atrocities committed around the world, the pain and suffering we can cause each other. But it is much closer to home than this. Any human being is capable of good or bad.

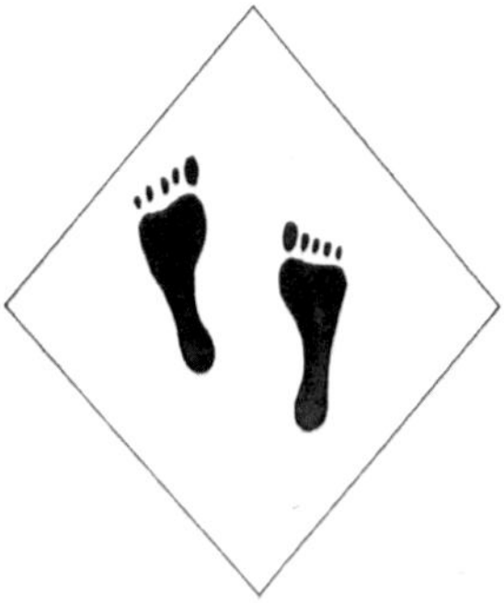

If you begin with the statement: 'I am capable of good and bad.'

How does this sit with you? Does it cause a reaction?

Yes, it can be difficult to both admit and accept this. Nonetheless, it is a fact and a truth – proven beyond doubt.

Do not bury your head in the sand nor seek justification of this. Your choice - if you are Being Omni, then your body will provide you with the correct answers: change, grow or stay as you are!

We are actually a mix of half and half: good thoughts and bad thoughts. Instead of denying your other side, Being Omni can teach you how to only live within your moments. We are *moving from thinking to feeling*; we are moving away from the mindsets of having to be good and avoiding the bad so neither good nor bad can hold any sway.

*****

The Crossroad

Duality then keeps us crucified by how far we have polarised the opposites of the things we believe in:

Love ---- Hate	Good ---- Bad
God ---- Devil	Light ---- Dark

We stand in the middle with the existence of each either side. This dichotomy means we are forever at a crossroad. We put ourselves upon the cross of suffering and indecision so that we end up crucifying ourselves daily.

Mind

Being pulled this way ~ Right O Left ~ Trying to avoid

Duality

Good ~ Right Left ~ Wrong

Choice

Trying to decide

Crossroads

Crucified

Not

in

the

nows

We are taught to gravitate towards God and avoid the Devil like the plague. This self-crucifixion has been our norm for a long time. *Duality* separates us from doing and being. Instead, it encourages us to live more within our minds where procrastination and indecision are masters!

∞

Choice and the endless dance of, Shall I? Shan't I?

Our domestication, our upbringing, the society in which we live, the media we absorb and many other things are there to keep a continual state of imbalance within your mind and body. It is the endless dance of the *Shall I? Shan't I?* saga within us.

When we refer to ourselves in the first person we use 'I'. For a moment, can you consider your inner dialogue and also what you say to others. It seems there is an 'I' in pretty much everything we think and say.

- o I am...
- o I know...
- o I will...
- o I won't...
- o I am no good at...
- o I am special...
- o I am no good in company...
- o I am too old...
- o I don't have this...
- o I want...
- o I need...
- o I am sorry...

BUT, the 'I' is a divided self. We are divided by our thinking within duality.

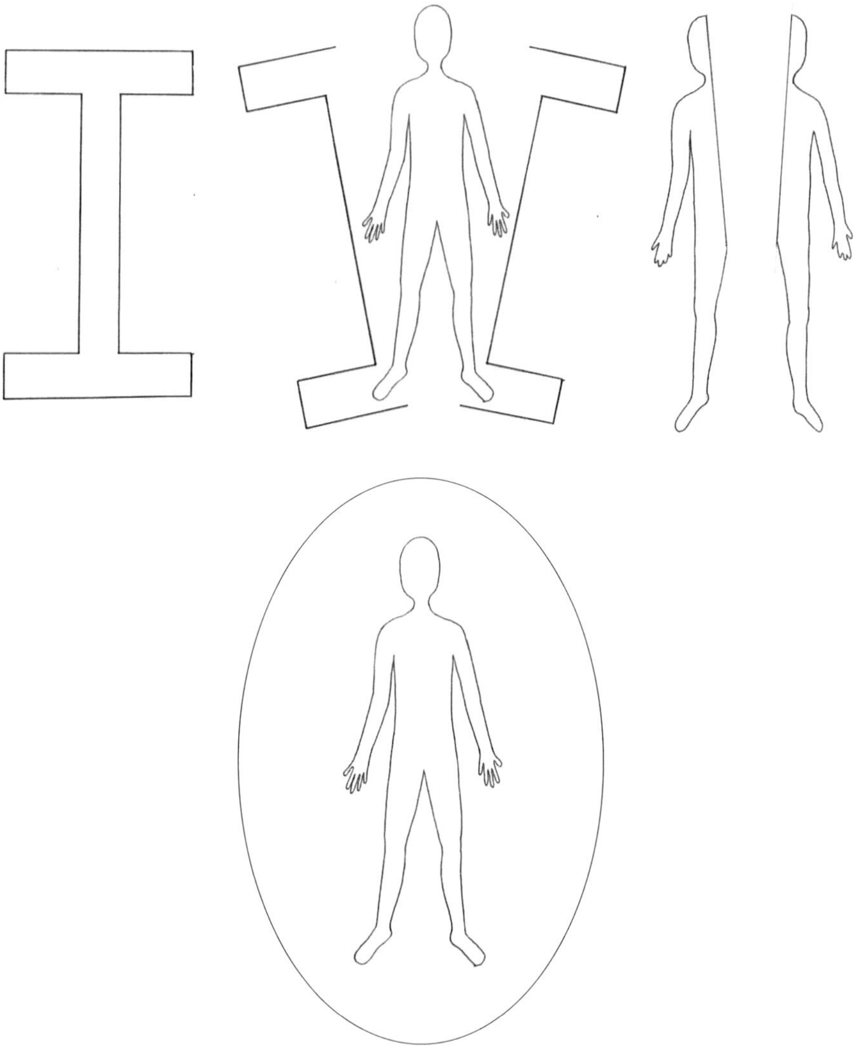

Consequently, while you are divided with right or wrong, you will remain weak and indecisive. Having choice and choosing again divides and weakens. Try and make decisions quickly, even major ones. Hesitation and indecisiveness not only weakens you but at the same time, strengths your reliability upon your mind. We are beguiled by what we think we know by how our minds let us feel.

People may do things that annoy you or wind you up. You can then choose to become angry with them or simply choose not to play their games. Everyone plays games with each other – stop right now.

It is not what others do or say, it is what you are doing and saying to yourself that is important. Being Omni helps you to minimise the reactions so they are no longer detrimental and you become more emotionally stable.

Our reactions come from many things...

- We react from known reactions – mindsets and past experiences.
- We react from our star sign traits.
- We react from a numerology stance.
- We react from a subconscious level.
- We react from a primate level (instant dislike).
- And, we react from a primal source.

When we have to choose something, it sometimes puts us in a dilemma, even into a spin of thoughts. We weigh up all the pros and cons and may dither about what to do for a long time. This does not do our bodies any good. We are torn and twisted by trying to decide what to do, what to buy, who to see and so on. We are effectively tormenting our selves (note the split in the word). This weakened state often means we agree to things or get easily persuaded even if we don't really want to do something. We feel obliged or guilty for saying no and end up going against what we really want to do. Whilst this goes on, we get more and more indecisive and hesitant and lose the plot allowing fear to take hold. If you can learn to decide quickly, even if it turns out to be the wrong choice, you will get help from any number of unexpected sources.

F-E-A-R can be used either way here:
Forget Everything And Run or Face Everything And Rise.
The choice is yours.

What to do? No matter if it's a new job, new house, new partner or what to buy in the shops, the secret is just to do.

Oh No! I have recently moved and I hate my new house/home (which word feels better, house or home?). Is the house going to kill you? That's the worst-case scenario. You may not like it or may feel uncomfortable there, but are you powerless? You have chosen to stress and worry about the house. You have chosen to torture yourself - no one else is doing this.

Start to change one room at a time and only one. Acceptance of the moment please, unless it is life-threatening. Acceptance helps to slow down the amount of stress. The rule is you can only change yourself and how you think, feel and react to things within your life and what is happening in your life. So, decorate one room. But, 'I have no money'. Wrong, everything we need is nearly always to hand. Move from a helpless state to a doing one, even if it is just an inexpensive throw to cover something. The next visitor may well have pots of paint lying around. *Trust.*

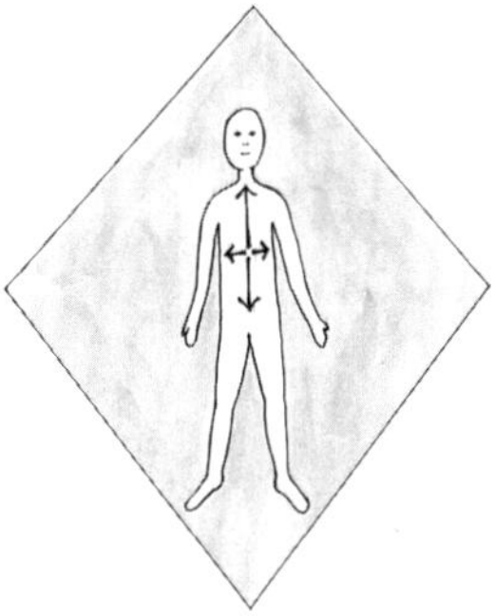

Listen to your body's responses to your questions – lean forward okay, lean backward not okay.

You have the magic within ready and willing to help you. Why? Because if you are all right, it is all right too. It cannot help whilst you are flapping about like a wounded bird. Either choose or forget about choosing anything and get on with your life. From now on you are going to learn to trust yourself and only yourself.

When bad things happen to us, we mostly get stuck in a thought process of 'Why did this happen?' and 'Who is responsible?' Today, we are in a culture of blame. It's always someone else that causes the problem. From family life to work and social interactions, it's them not me; it's all their fault, never mine. Can you let it go?

Take appropriate action and move on ~ good will always come out of a bad event. You may not agree with this but nevertheless, it's true. Bad things happen to create change because usually we are so reluctant to do so. Events are then set in place to force a change. Please take note of signs and warnings that are trying to help you.

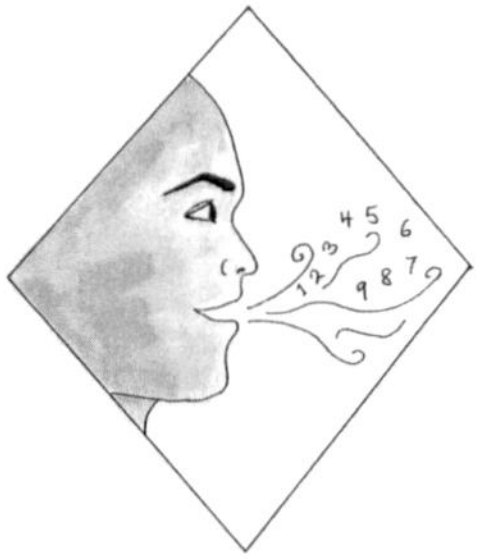

◊ *Stop – breathe – take control. No matter what the problem is, or how difficult it is to decide something, stop and put it on hold and begin to take the first few steps of Being Omni.*

Be in Omni which will then allow the answers or solutions to present themselves.

> *"Use of the Omni breathing and sensing through my body and feet really does seem to restore calm. Any decision to make seems much less important and a way forward can just happen after using the steps."*
>
> *Jenny Underhill*

∞

Time to Choose ~ Old or New?

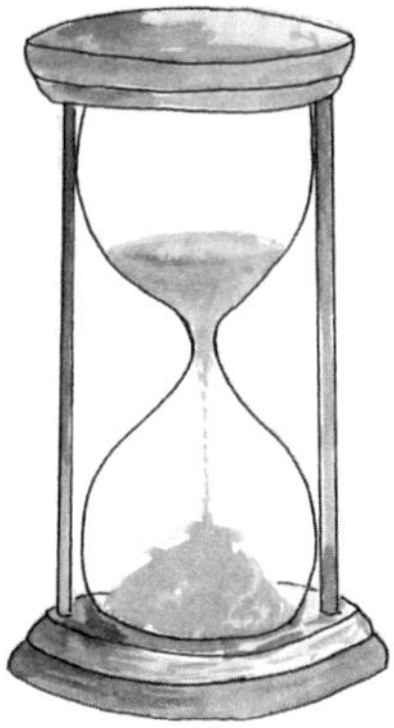

Being Omni gives us choice back. It gives us the power to choose. Of course, we are all *led* to believe we have choice and freedom in the things we say and do. But this is part of the illusion. In truth, we are funnelled and domesticated and directed hither and thither constantly. Once you truly begin to know yourself and assemble your whole being in the body's correct time and space, then you will become you and not what the mind has created. Knowing your true self is the very first lesson in oneness.

When you are practising the steps, you will be able to use your body's *yes* – *no* answering mechanisms. Please remember your body lives in real earth time. It also does not have any agendas or know rights or wrongs. These belong solely to your mind. This does not mean you will care any less instead your being is fully aware and totally compatible with all things.

There are many 'old' ways of being which lead us to doubt in the self and continually reinforce the need to wear the masks that hide or distort who we truly are.

*****

Externals

Part of the reason we have become this way is because we have looked outside of ourselves for answers. Let's call this, a belief in externals. Externals can be *anything* outside of you: religion, society, other people. There are far too many things to write here, but our faiths and beliefs have predominantly been in externals. People have always wanted and needed something to guide them, rules to follow, something to feel a part of – to be connected to and reliant upon. In part, we believe something else is greater which is essentially giving over our power to something other than the self.

Many years ago, when my journey on a psychic level began, I attended a spiritual meeting. The medium at the time said an opening prayer asking for all to be taken into the light and ascend to heaven or something of the like. This is, more or less, the same with all religions: follow my rules and I will save you. I sat there listening and as I looked into the corners of the room, at those in spirit form that dwell or are stuck in between worlds, dimensions and times, I could see that they were afraid of the light. These were the ones who have never known what it is like to be loved, cared for, and nourished by another. All they know is the darkness of their inner souls. These were never helped.

And at this moment in time, although my knowledge of religions is not worldly, in my Omni way, I feel and sense what is right for me and these kinds of external beliefs do not help all.

We also grow up following what our parents believe in for a time or until we reach an age where we begin to question and seek our own answers. But even then, the information we find does not lead to the truth, it always leads to someone else's beliefs or truths.

How many beliefs do you actually have? What do you believe in?

Journal opportunity ~ Make a list of your beliefs, please. This will take longer than one day and should be added to as and when.

The one place we never or rarely look is within. Even if you do, the true you is shrouded by so many masks, roles, beliefs and illusions that you have created, it is hard to find the real you.

Being Omni gives you a chance to evolve and to be the creative being you truly are. Shackles away, out of the mud, turn out the light and just be. It is all about becoming you...

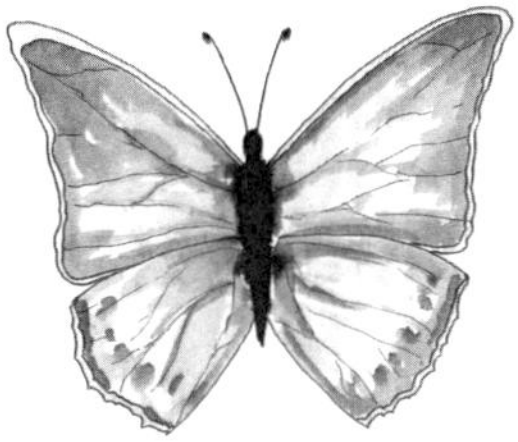

◊ *Omni is not a belief system. It does not have allegiance to anything else.The only beliefs are self belief and belief in the self's processes.*

*****

The Pecking Order

It is hard to ignore the pecking order that runs or governs our living. The pyramid of power has ruled us from the beginning. In very simple terms, it is one person at the top, two just below who want the top position at any cost, three below them who have aspirations but not the total ruthlessness, hence people who are the bullies and do all the dirty work. Then we have two more sections of the masses who believe in the system one hundred percent, and then a small lower group who are unhappy at things but do not have the power to create change. They moan and groan a lot, postulating and speculating, but never really make an impact.

The pecking order belongs in the age of the dinosaurs!

Omni helps you *evolve* beyond this.

There is a point in everyone's consciousness that we have yet to reach. This is when we strip away beliefs, faiths, hierarchies and masks from our thinking. Then we begin to see that we are all just human beings. Being Omni starts a levelling process so the old pecking order syndrome reduces, along with the primal needs and ultimately, the primate survival instincts. When these reduce enough, we can establish a much cleaner consciousness.

Our primate self or part is still very much to do with the pecking order. Those above and below you will perpetually tease or say or do things that upset or annoy you, causing your displacement in the pecking order so they can win.

The pecking order within each of us needs to be understood and then altered to suit our new awareness of the present moments. This system is not something directly under conscious control but by using the Omni steps, you can begin to master and control your responses to it. In other words, how you choose to react.

◊ *When you are practising the Omni steps, you and your body both evolve, reducing the effect of these so you actually grow and develop and begin to live.*

*****

Domestication and Masks

Domestication is also entrenched in our current way of being and existing and part of the process of self-domestication is that we learn to adopt different masks. Most of us wear masks for every one we know. We adopt these masks because we are taught roles for each situation in our lives. The role of mother, friend, teacher, wife, brother, colleague and it goes on and on.

I can say with absolute certainty very few people actually know themselves. And it is not your fault or anyone else's for that matter. When we were born, we were not given a life manual, nor was anyone else. Our parents learnt from their parents and all those around them with no-one knowing the real truth in how to be or act or behave.

Our true self, the real self, hides under all the masks, roles and illusions each of us have created to get us through things and to cope with life. Without exception, everyone has done this.

◊ *Free yourself from the mind's version of you and find yourself – the true you.*

If you use Being Omni a few times every day, the number of roles you have adopted for every person and situation you know, will reduce bit by bit. You will still be you but the real you. You can tell this is happening as friends will either increase or diminish as you have taken off the mask and no longer play that role for them.

*****

Truth or Illusion

No one has ever really been told the truth, but in Omni living *you become the truth.* Your truth at first but as you progress with Omni, the common truths become more apparent.

Nothing that has gone before prepares you for the nows and the moments but Omni lets you live within every new moment that occurs for you. Nothing in the future is ever real; it's only what your thoughts can conjure up or what your expectation of things are – these only exist as thoughts and can *never be real.*

So, you can see, finding yourself may seem very complex while limited to words and thinking. There is a much easier way once you begin to live in your here and nows which gives you access to more real and true time, and proper moments.

◊ *The present is the only time that really exists.*

Consider this for a moment: no other time really exists as they are all part of the illusions of the mind. Being Omni is all about learning 'how' to live in the present and in doing so, you can connect to your reality – the reality of who you are, where you are and what is happening at that moment.

This is the *only* time that change can actually happen.

∞

Learning to stick with reality of your moments

We live in a world where time seems important to many. We also live *on* a world with its seasons and times of change: four times a year for everybody. The earth has its own time relative to these seasons. A long time ago, humans fitted into this cycle - migrating with each season, going north in the early summer until they reached a temperate climate that suited them and moving in a figure of eight pattern south as the weather changed, going where the food trail was (but not eating everything in sight!). They always just took what they needed and left some for other travellers. They also followed (perhaps without knowing) Venus and her dance as she touched the earth's fields every so often.

Time is always flowing and moving forwards according to the seasons, nature and the weather. Yet today we have mostly lost this way of being and living, and before someone says there are tribes out there that do, they now only live in a tenth of the area they need to do this properly. We have stepped out of this natural cycle of time flowing and moving and learnt to live in the mind's version of time or mind time and this has very little connection to real or true time.

*****

What is mind time?

We have frequently referred to mind time throughout the different sections of this book, but what is it? How can we explain it in more detail?

We mentioned earlier about how the mind and our thoughts and thinking can work – well, this is inextricably linked with time. It's about how we view it, how we use it, why it is so very precious to us and yet, for many, how time seems to be speeding up. We obsess over never having enough time. Think about how often you hear this or how often you say or think this – 'There is never enough time.' We use time as an excuse and waste it...continually.

The reason everything seems to be speeding up and it feels like we are always running out of time is because we exist in mind time. Mind time is the illusion. It is the opposite of real time or reality or the present flowing moments. We have come live within our mind's view of time and the things that happen to us within timed events and stages of our lives. We are completely detached from real time itself - and this is not living at all!

The following quote from Alan Watts[7] sums this up perfectly: "We are living in a culture entirely hypnotized by the illusion of time, in which the so-called present moment is felt as nothing but an infinitesimal hairline between a causative past

---

[7] Alan Wilson Watts was a British philosopher, writer, and speaker, who was one of the first to interpret Eastern wisdom for a Western audience.

and an absorbingly important future. We have no present. Our consciousness is almost completely preoccupied with memory and expectation. We do not realize that there never was, is, nor will be any other experience than present experience. We are therefore out of touch with reality."

This means that you never notice the moments, the nows as they come and go. Yet in reality, in real time, there is only ever the nows and the moments you are in. Everything else is your mind's illusion of time, distorted by living within your past, and the dreams and illusions of your future.

- ◊ *When you are enjoying something, and are totally absorbed in that task, time is different. Everything flows properly. You are fully engaged in the moments. Nothing else matters during this time. We become timeless and so does the world around us.*

Just have a look at some common every day occurrences, and you can see how you have used time so far and how you are predominantly existing in mind time. If you are running late for a meeting and rushing off to get there – is time fast or slow? What about when you are waiting for a bus or a friend to meet you or are stuck in a queue – does time speed up or drag? If you are bored and have heard it all before, time slowly passes. On the other hand, if you're interested and enjoying something, time seems to be fine. Yet, all around you time flows at the normal rate – fact.

Try and make a distinction between these if you can – it will free up ninety percent of your mind. You could control your time much better if you want to by how *you* think and not how your mind wants you to think. By becoming more and more aware of this and by practising the Omni steps, it will not only help you to distinguish between these different times but will help you access the reality of your moments more and more and give you more actual time.

What is the only true time that really exists?

NOW

But how long does a now last? And is there always another one?

Humans and their thoughts always get stuck in certain types of nows. When something good or bad happens, it sticks in our minds. If you think of your mind as a hard drive or disc, a scratch can cover a few sections. Bad experiences scar or scratch the hard drive of memories, making it easier to go back to that memory and replay it. This only deepens the scratch. Good events don't do this, instead they drift off to a far corner of our consciousness and are much harder to find and replay.

Using Omni helps us become unstuck and allows us to be more in the present moments as well as giving us a new hard drive whenever we want!

Eckhart Tolle wrote some good books on the power of now, but we must recognise that a now is a singular event that only lasts a few seconds or even a minute but is gone in a flash. It is always followed by a gap and then another now. The length of a now and the gap between is completely under your control. Usually, when we experience the gaps, our minds kick in and then they get filled with thoughts. This is how the distance between the nows can be rather large.

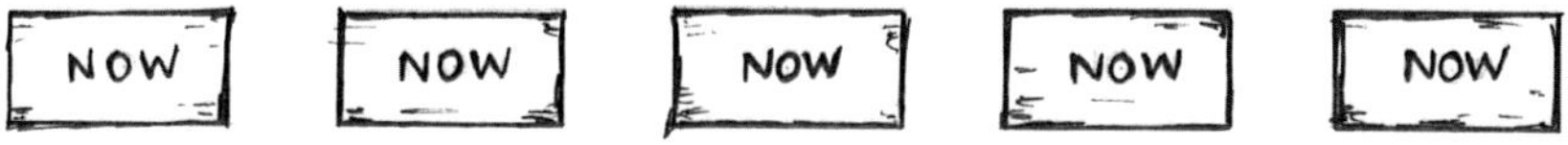

Yet when a person begins to live in their nows, they begin to synchronously flow from one to another, avoiding the gaps in between the nows.

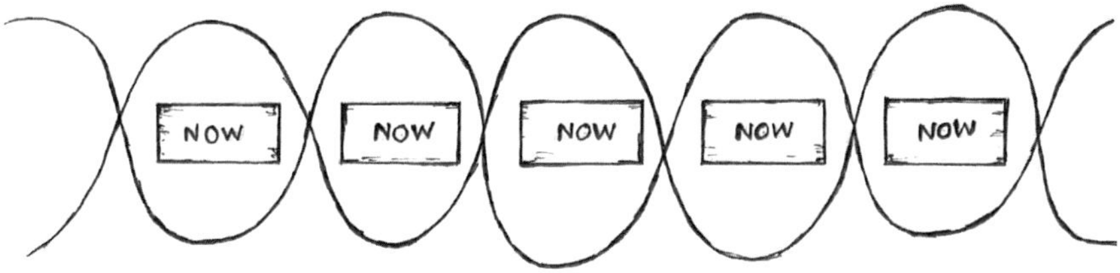

And as far as I know, five to seven nows make a moment and when you move through the levels of Being Omni, you do not have nows but flowing moments of living and being in a wonderful world.

But to start us off, we begin with a now and your awareness of that now and learn how to use your body in real time.

Our external awareness is connected to the reality around a person: the firmness of your footing on the floor you are standing upon, and our inner awareness is about the weight your body is exerting upon the floor. This is actually affected by the different moods and thoughts you experience yet the floor remains the same firmness. The air you are breathing in may be cold but it carries a lot of things that your body senses via smell and taste. Therefore, we can *sense* reality and we can *feel* where it interacts with our body. We also hear, we see, we smell, and taste what is externally real around us. But even before we begin to digest this information, the mind alters it to suit what it thinks you need to know right now.

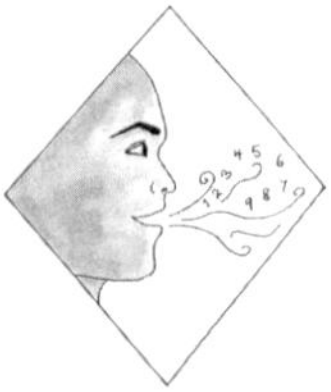

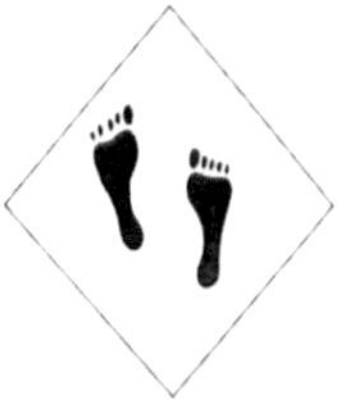

Once you have mastered sensing and feeling alongside controlled breathing, your awareness of the nows and your moments increases. This means you are no longer a prisoner of old or new mind times – you are completely free and in real time at last! You have finally begun your journey, no longer dependent on anyone or anything else, and you are now free to evolve and use your true creativeness.

*****

A Moment

It really does not matter what you have done, nor does it matter what you think you might do. You can only do something in the moment you actually decide to. Yes, you can plan many things – go for a walk tomorrow, yet you miss out on the benefits of walking right now.

Nows and moments are the times of great power and the only time real and actual change can happen.

Silent Power by Stuart Wilde explains about how much power we give away to others and how we lose immense amounts of energy by putting our energy (thoughts) into future events. If your mind ever lands in your nows and moments, you will have anywhere between 75-95% of pure energy available to do anything.

Can I ask you to create a moment for yourself? It's not a big request, but a learning tool on your Omni journey. No matter what your present circumstance, a taken moment has tremendous value to each and every one of us. Stop whatever you are doing, find a comfortable place to either sit or lie down, and begin your first moments.

- ◊ *Pause and ask yourself the following, 'Are there any problems right now?'*

Wherever you are or whatever you are doing, try to do this every so often. It's not only a very quick reality check but it allows your body and mind to synchronise in real time. Mind and body at one. This allows the time and space that your mind and thoughts used to take up to reduce. This is where the less is more principle can become fully active in your life: less thoughts, less thinking = more you, more time and more space.

When we do this the first few times, our thoughts will present problems or issues that the mind carries along with it, but right here, right now there cannot be a problem nor an issue. Practise this and each time stillness within draws ever closer.

And many, many more things can happen in that moment. You could have a realisation, a revelation or epiphany, no pain, instant healing, a feeling of joy or happiness – so many things can happen in a moment. And I can almost guarantee only good happens in a moment. Why the word almost? Your mind will conjure up all sorts of things to spoil your moment. I cannot account for your thoughts, but I do know with absolute certainty, moments without the mind are truly wonderful and magical for anyone.

Please start to practise having a moment and do not close your eyes. In fact, become aware of what you can see. It does not matter if there is only a plain wall in front of you, absorb what you see. Meditation is a life saver for many. They rest, recover and enjoy their meditation and it is good for them. But on finishing the session, the real world awaits – your problems, worries and stresses have not diminished but you may be able to cope with things a little better. Moments give you so much more than this and the issues and problems and worries may well have improved. Wayne Dwyer states: *When you change the way you look at things, the things you look at change.* A powerful set of words. In a moment taken properly, you change for your own self-betterment.

> *"In Being Omni, I am whole and I can be fully myself in this moment, free and un-constricted by any false mental cages that have at times seemed like a prison. In Being Omni, there is no box around me. I can flow through the moments in a situation with inner knowing that the steps and the moves I choose to make are the right ones."*
>
> *Thoby Davis*

I cannot say truly that I know what will happen when people take or make these steps, but I do know that when you actually begin to embrace the reality of your moments, the energy part comes alive. Omni is all about the reality of your moments - not what your thoughts of reality are! This is a journey that humans have never taken. The thoughts or images the mind creates and sustains, make up the illusion of you and your daily life.

Life is a singular word here, living is a real-time word, world and reality.

Houston, we have a problem! It's called thinking and most people cannot stop it.

What are your solutions?

You can stick with thinking or try Being Omni. Feel ~ sense ~ do ~ be ~ aware ~ live now. There's a heck of a difference. You have spent a lifetime getting to this point, so the old you, your old ways, habits, routines and beliefs will keep dragging you back. This really does take effort and practice and you have to decide if you want to or if it's worth it to you. In one way it is a huge step but Being Omni is a safe and easy way to do this. The steps will help you as you battle your mind and old self which you hide within.

∞

Life is for Living

Of course, it is wonderful to experience and create stillness and balance within your moments, but life doesn't necessarily happen on an even keel. It is full of ups and downs. We are human and would not learn very much if we did not experience the full extent of what life has to offer. After all, life is for living.

However, it is how these highs and lows affect us and how we react to them that can cause us problems. Up until now, our moods change drastically as we oscillate between these peaks and troughs. If something good happens, we feel elated and overjoyed. And on the other side, when something bad happens we crash into depression and despair. When we live like this, our emotions are in charge and we are constantly reacting to any situation or person.

If someone says or does something to upset you, how long do you remain hurt? When someone annoys you and you become angry, regardless of whether you say anything or not at the time, what happens to that anger? If it stays within you, it begins to eat away inside of you. In most cases, the things that annoy us build up bit by bit and eventually we blow our stack. We are like volcanoes in this way and it can be something minor that eventually leads us to blow our tops. The fact that built up anger or stress can resurface at any time means that you have been carrying it around with you for the whole time. It's like carrying baggage you didn't even realise you had.

Remember that bad events or experiences leave scratches all over your hard drive. The more these memories are replayed or revisited in your mind, the deeper the scratch gets and the more it has power to influence your present reactions and decisions. In this way, our reactions are often extreme and, through our own choice and participation, we stay on the roller coaster.

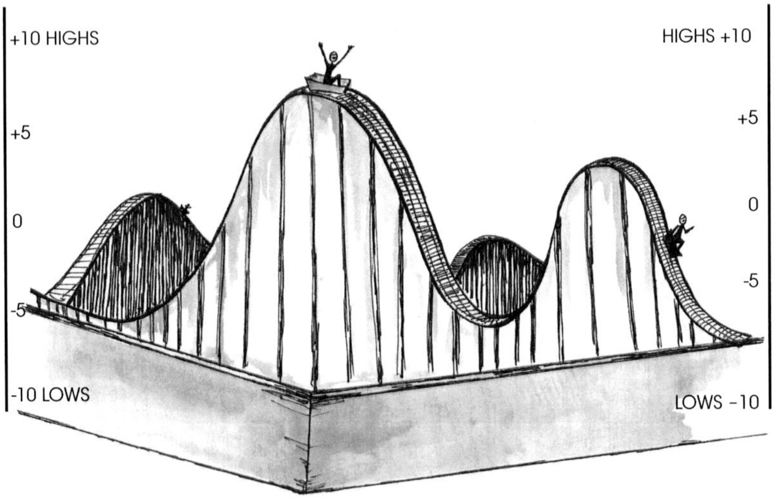

We have to look at two things here. One, a fact: no one else can make you angry. You actually choose and decide to become angry at this person because they say or do something you don't like or approve of. The second thing is, what does anger or becoming angry do to your physical body and your emotions?

When held within these two, knots of tension happen usually in the first part of your stomach. A tightness or knot or lump can be felt. Tension and inner stresses are fed by the anger and tighten up and it may also affect your breathing. In truth, all our negative emotions harm different parts of the body.

This gap between the highs and lows needs to lessen so that instead it becomes more gentle ups and downs. There is nothing wrong with being overjoyed but it is how high you go, and if something happens to knock you out of this high, it's a long way down.

Try and stay within +5 and -5 area (the safe-zone). If you find yourself dipping below -5 take action. Try the Omni steps or busy yourself. You may not feel like it but it will stop the fall and allow you to rise. We can find a simple see-saw balance that allows us to be ourselves. Yes, we can still get angry and even shout, but if you use the steps you are able to move the see-saw in a conscious way. This allows the anger to disperse and fade away quickly and easily so you can reset and stop harming your body. And you have begun not to let go of things (this is a pretence) but to live in your nows and moments where you are aware and present and totally compatible to everything else in your world and universe.

Some reactions come unbidden. These are from the primate and primal minds where we have an instant like or dislike of a place or person. These reactions require no thinking but are based on the energy of what you are encountering at that time. As this happens, consciously move into your here and nows right away through breathing and sensing. This reduces the influence of the primal and primate parts of you and lets you begin to use your own evolutionary journey of whole body and whole mind.

> *"Being Omni is a state of being which could be described as being alert, flowful, focussed and in-the-zone but perhaps even these descriptions fall somewhat short. For example, it is possible to be in an Omni state and feel anger. It is possible to be in an Omni state and feel sadness, perhaps even fear. For sometimes these emotions are what is required in a given situation...however, in Omni these emotions will not last long and can be recognised for what they are – simply the mind's reactions to said situation and are fleeting."*
>
> *Thoby Davis*

∞

Reset methods

As you move more and more into Being Omni, the need to look after and protect yourself should grow less and less. But every now and then, we could all use a reset. The following exercises work alongside the steps and will definitely help if you get a little thrown off balance.

*****

Cook's-Hook-Up

During some of the healing therapies I teach, we use what is called *Cook's Hook Up*. It can be used as basic protection from other people's negative thoughts and energies but also works to bring your energy part back in sync with your body. It is a fantastic reset tool which helps mind, body and energy part rebalance.

Try it first by sitting down. You cross one ankle over the other. Left or right, it doesn't matter a minute. Then place your hands together, crossing them so your palms are facing. Interlock your fingers and either loop your hands back to your chest area or let your hands rest on your lap.

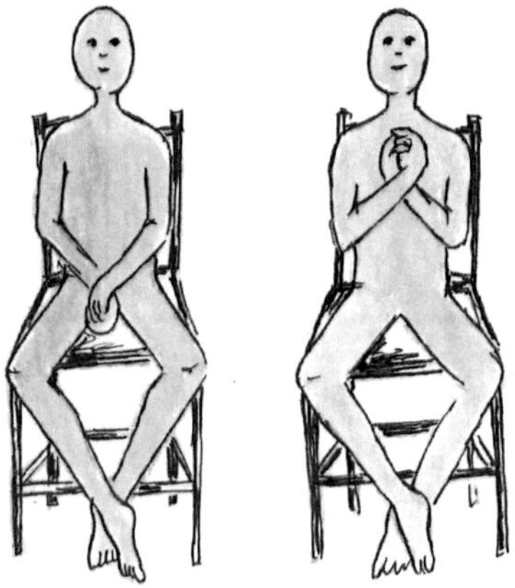

Using your body this way, creates a figure of eight: the symbol of infinity. Once you have had a go at the seated one, try it standing up. It is always worthwhile experimenting with this. It's quick and easy to do wherever you are.

Even though we are using the steps and Being Omni, sometimes something will happen from an external source that will flip you out of it. This can be traumatic to say the least. One minute you are feeling good and safe and progressing, then bang, back into vulnerability and uncertainty and worse than before as you may feel totally exposed. This is a good time for Cook's Hook Up! And, at the same time, start Step One and complete a breathing cycle.

*****

The Circumpunct

Another useful tool is the circumpunct. When you feel the need to reset, draw a circumpunct (circle with dot) on a piece of paper and place a finger upon the dot or your hand over the image. This helps you immediately reset energy-wise.

You could try this variation too. Using your finger, draw an imaginary one on your palm – the circle is always created first and then the dot. Or even draw one in water or sand.

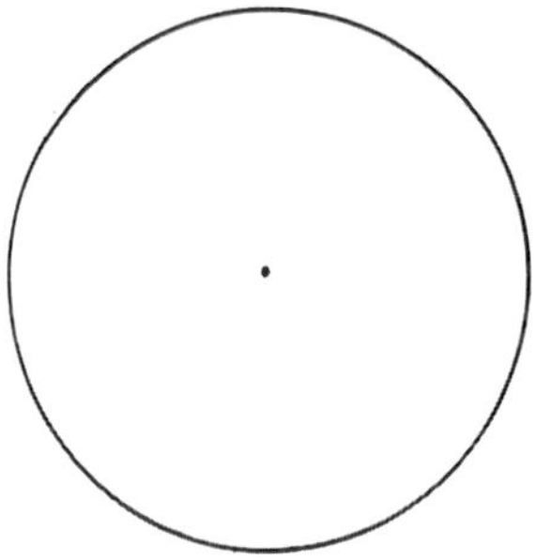

*****

Using your imagination

What does the word imagination mean? For myself, I think of something or someone and at the same time I may see a picture within my mind. It is the ability to see an image within your mind's eye and is something that everyone can do. It might require plenty of practising but it is well worth this effort. Can you *image in* a picture of a tree? A lovely rose? Your front door? Have a go, please.

However, imagination cuts both ways. If you are looking ahead to say a job interview, your imagination may go into overdrive and create all sorts of bad scenarios or things that can go wrong for you. On the other hand, it is also capable of creating a wonderful scenario of a perfect interview and a job offer. These are associated with the mind's versions of our future *what ifs*.

Imagination is linked to a part of us separate from the mind. A part that does not know right from wrong. It is a power source that can make things manifest or happen. Most people tap into this on a daily basis with their normal everyday thinking. Remember the chapter on thoughts and thinking - oh the roads will be busy, and they are. Again, the other side is seeing them clear and having an easy journey.

Being Omni enables you to tap into these extra, unused abilities. Imagination and visualisation are two of these abilities that we all have, and these provide a link from the real you to the world of energy within everyone.

Using imagination and visualisation in the following ways will help you in your everyday life. They help by protecting you from negative energies and, if you have an illness, enable you to utilise your body's own healing capacity.

*****

The Daisy

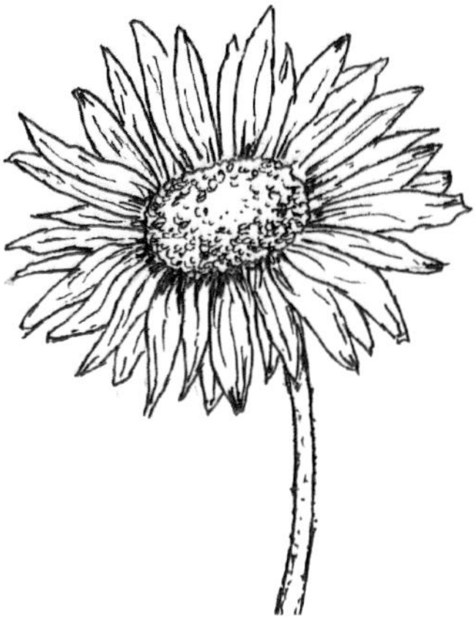

Just for a moment I would like you to use your imagination to create an image of a daisy. When you have the image, try and hold it in your mind's eye.

What details can you see? The head of a daisy? Delicate, curling white petals and maybe a yellow centre? Does it have a stem? What shape or length is it? Does the stem go into the ground? And are there some thin, fine roots under the earth?

Try and build up a complete picture, and then think about becoming that daisy...

Now try and look at the whole picture in your mind; the complete daisy and its surroundings.

This represents you as you are right now.

How straight is the stem?
Which way is the head of your daisy facing?
How deep are the roots?
Is your daisy fully or only partially open?

Take note of how you are feeling right now.

Go back to the image of your daisy, and visualise gentle rain falling on it, washing each petal, then running down the stem and into the earth. Now shift into an image and begin visualising warm sunshine radiating down onto your daisy. After a while, the two things (imagination and visualisation) combine and begin to work as one, not from your thoughts nor mind but from an energy centre. And by using the image of your daisy, it will help strengthen your link to your inner mind where you can start to make simple but easy changes that benefit you in many ways.

Now, how do you feel?

*****

A Tree's Seasons

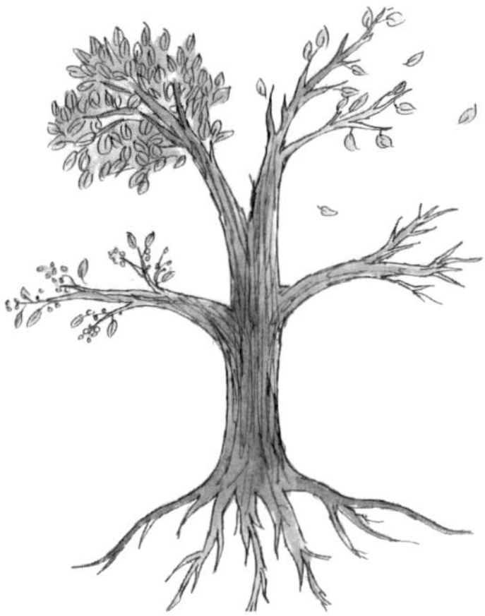

Once you have had a few goes with imagining a daisy, try it now with your tree.

When you *imagine* a picture of a tree, it's good to check whether it is one that is free of the mind's thoughts and associated feelings. Usually, when I ask people to imagine a picture of a tree, they will always come up with a mind-orientated version of a strong healthy tree, an oak perhaps, because that is what the mind creates in response to being asked. Clear that image away and try again.

You might see a picture of a tree that's not in its prime or is misshapen in some way or another. This represents you within that moment.

Let's say for example, it's April and the buds on most of the trees in my garden have yet to open. If my image is of a tree in full bloom, I know it is out of season. I look at the picture again and imagine a breeze or gentle rain and the image changes. This is using visualisation to bring the image to life.

My tree image has changed and is now in full summer so I imagine and visualise it moving into autumn. The leaves turn yellows and browns, great winds and rain come along and blow the leaves away and they begin their cycle of feeding the next tree - natural recycling at its best! Then I begin to see it in midwinter where all is quiet and cold and still. Just as it settles here, I see spring beginning and little buds starting to form. And now, I'm back in April. This exercise aligns me with the correct times and seasons of the earth.

Along with imagining this, my body also went through some decluttering. The leaves being blown away equals my worries and fears fading away. My body rested while I imagined my tree in mid-winter and new life began to flow as the sap rose in the tree, so my body is refreshed too.

All I can do is ask you to try this and note what happens to your body and mind before, during and after it.

Imagination and visualisation can become great tools for your self-benefit.

*****

Acupressure points

Top lip

Throughout our bodies are nerve plexus points. Some of these are connectors where other nerve lines branch off and around some of these are meridian nodal points. Acupuncture and acupressure therapists both tap into these; one with needles, the other with gentle pressure and movements. Both therapies help in some ways, yet you can use basic acupressure ones on yourself. Please be gentle as you begin to practise these.

Place your index finger on your top lip right in the centre (there's usually a dip here to help you locate it) and apply a small amount of pressure. As you do, you should take in an involuntary breath. Then gently push upwards towards nose and hold a steady but gentle amount of pressure.

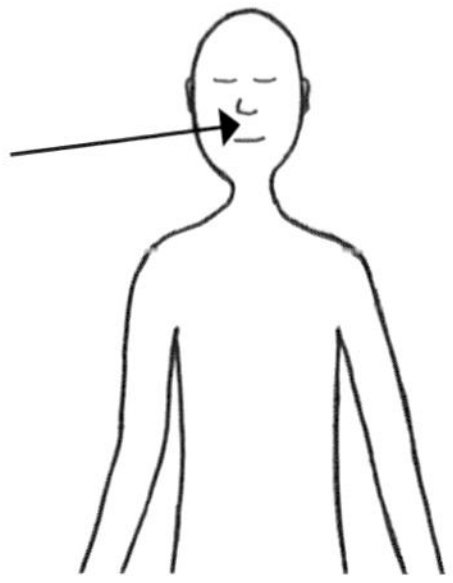

This will help you rebalance and settle.

Thymus

Next to practise on is your thymus. It is said by many to be redundant after a certain age which is true but the energy counterpart is very much alive and, in most cases, working flat out.

The thymus is part of our primal-primate systems and to do with our safety. It's part of the flight or fight survival system: when in danger we either run away or stand and fight. Yet it has little use in today's world. That's not to say it's inactive, it's actually over-active. If you watch TV programmes or the news, they are all geared up to make you respond. You will have some sort of thoughts about what you are seeing and hearing that cause the thymus counterpart to send a message to the adrenals to begin to pump out adrenaline into your blood stream. This happens quite often during your day without you even realising. Something happens, you react and respond and this sets of a chain of events within your body. For some people they become full of unused adrenaline. An easy way to check this is to grasp your upper arm and squeeze. If it feels tender or there are any sore spots, then it may well be full of decaying adrenaline and blocking up other systems within your arm and body.

When I see clients for various healing and treatments, I would often make their next appointment a trip to the leisure centre to go swimming. This is not the answer to all problems but if done on a regular basis, swimming clears the adrenaline from your arms and legs and in general you will get healthier.

Today's world is fast-paced and designed to wind you up, this is why Being Omni is a life saver.

Another way to prevent your system flooding with adrenaline is to use the acupressure thymus point. Find the centre of your sternum (breastbone), use two fingers and press this area gently. Apply a small amount of pressure as it may feel tender, hold the pressure and do not increase it. Just hold the pressure until tenderness reduces. Then apply a little more pressure and the same again. Doing this twice will turn off the auto alarm of fight or flight.

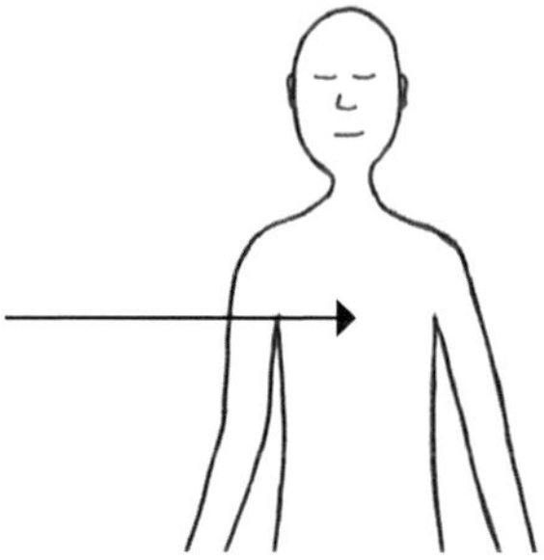

Why do we need Omni?

For so many of us, the pace of life is out of control. Just consider now how your days go. Work? Home? Social life? Holidays? Do your days become weeks and those become years? Somehow you have lost months, leading the life you believe you should.

Stop.

Be honest in your personal appraisal of your daily life please. And depending on your answer, and if your life is ok and you are sure, then that is fine.

But please read and re-read through this book and when you begin to truly understand and you have learnt to listen to your body, you may well begin to have a change of mind.

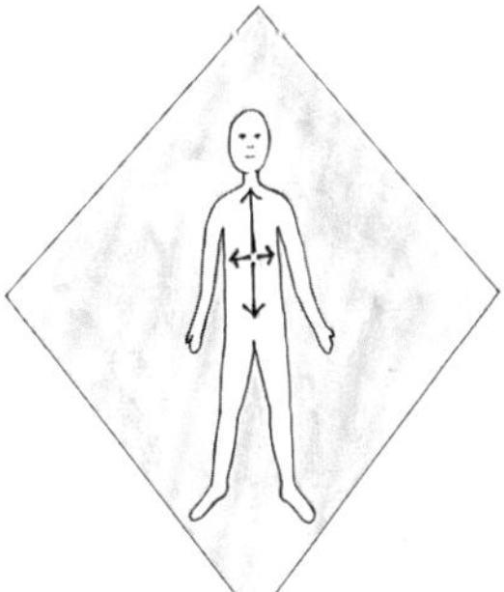

Think about making some little changes to your lifestyle and start Being Omni in small ways. For myself, it really does help my daily life. I have two daughters and one grandson who I believe will be helped as life changes for us all. There is no place you can run off to, build a bunker or live on an island safe and sound. These changes not only affect human life, but all life, the seasons, nature and the core of the earth.

I have been a great observer of people all my life and spent many a time wandering about the place, watching the early morning people rushing off to work in their cars, to people working in the shops and the shoppers all in a rush, nobody really aware of their moments as their minds are always somewhere else.

◊ *The speed of life does not give us the time to appreciate our actual lives.*

On one particular trip, I was visiting various places with friends. Heading along the busy motorways showed that we all just dash from one place to another. It was a Friday, a day when lots of people go off for a rest in their holiday homes to recuperate. It's sad but I doubted if they really do this because they are already thinking ahead to work next week. Most people have learnt to live in mind time, thinking ahead and never in real time, so I likened all this to people being on hamster wheels: home one, work one, social time one – all on an endless cycle. We then went to Ely Cathedral and again lots of people were walking around taking pictures looking at the magnificent building, buying gifts for others and then off for lunch and then next place and so on, endlessly doing the same sort of things but never really living. This pattern of living can be seen anywhere!

The speed of life is also very much driven by events and the media. There are people somewhere who benefit from us being controlled and manipulated (self-domestication also). Life for many has become a huge roller-coaster with highs and lows dominating our daily, weekly, yearly lives - many may have dropped out of society because it has become so sick, yet they are ostracised and pummelled from pillar to post. We need to ask ourselves why are we still being controlled by our primal instincts and primate behaviourisms, and why are we still held tightly within the pecking order?

Recent gruesome happenings testify to this. Mass globalisation is taking place. There are many people now needing a safe place to live and be. But this attracts the sort of people who bully and dominate those seeking sanctuary. There are more and more areas of conflict and trouble and strife are much closer to home now, and even within some people reading this. Their minds may still be split by duality and indecision within their thinking. These are all old, outdated ways of living and being that no longer serve us well.

Our world and our human consciousness has changed, and we have not. We can do wonderful things yet there is something missing in everybody's lives. Depression, stress and anxiety seem to have become the norm for many.

We have also been very lax in appreciating the world around us and how much we just take from it, and never put anything back apart from sewage and rubbish. We are now beginning to fill the once pristine areas in our planet with pollution and fill outer-space with debris, littering the earth's immediate air space.

Have we reached a point of no return?

Life is fluid and moving constantly. Humans like routines, fixed things, patterns and have become creatures of habit, resisting change at all cost. Ever since we decided to remove ourselves from the food chain and begin to think and act like we are superior to all other species, we have lost our connection to evolution and the ability to create and use the magic within.

◊ *Omni is a natural state of being that has zero adverse effects upon you or anything else.*

Humans have many things to learn and little time to do so, but the first is to learn about ourselves. We are so much more that what we seem on the surface. We have far more abilities than we have ever realised nor are we restricted to just our human bodies. I do not seek to prove any of this, that is for each of you to do, not me!

Being Omni is about waking up and taking responsibility for your *self*, and the world you live upon, not to change the world but to help us begin to change. It is the way to personal freedom and growth.

Of course, a lot depends on whether you want to make changes and embrace the Omni way of being. You can stay exactly the same - staying in the same routines, habits and old ways of living, or you can use Omni to start a process of self-betterment.

It not only helps you but also everyone around you, without any effort on your part.

*****

The Evolution Within

It's also a great step towards the evolution within as it leads to being able to reduce your primal and primate reactions and actions that have been with us since the beginning. Being Omni will help us begin a new evolutionary process. It's a way of being a whole person where body and mind function together, alongside of the energy counterpart that has been adrift for a long time.

◊ *Our humanness is so important because it is the only form in which change and transformation can take place.*

Change and evolution are an inextricable part of all life. And this is only ever possible in our human form as we are today. It requires us just to be ourselves, not something else. Robert is just Robert with all his foibles, idiosyncrasies, rights and wrongs. But he is a human being first and foremost and true acceptance of this allows the space for change to happen. He will not turn into a great, god-like being, nor will he fly through the air. Yet he will have mastered time and space, so distance from one place to another is of no matter. He will still have thoughts, feelings and reactions to the world around him but if he becomes angry at someone or something, it is very short lived. I do hope you can bear with my words and my writings and practise the parts of knowing your own truths.

This is where Being Omni helps ~ it gives you a sense of being and allows you to re-establish evolution within.

◊ *Omni = evolution without the need for revolution ~ change without change (in our humanness)*

*****

Commonality

~ Omni is of Latin origin meaning ALL ~

There is always hope for the future of humankind and the simplicity of Being Omni is one proper step forwards into being our real selves, as individuals at first but as Omni is contagious (in a good way), it leads to commonality ~ unity and harmony for all.

The way humanity has developed means we are born and grow up in a world which leads to a separateness in our living. Our interactions with other people are at a distance, and each encounter leaves us at a bit of a loss of self and inner energy. Many people will disagree with these words and all I ask is that you stop and look at your own interactions with others. As a race or species, we have come a long way but the one thing we do not yet know is about ourselves, our individual selves. We have woven illusions and wear masks and play roles and games within every single interaction we have with others.

Omni is simple and it helps anyone extricate them *selves* (note the split) from this state of being into a state of living and being part of the world around them once again. We are still very much ruled by our primate and primitive selves especially in terms of how we react. The steps help everyone rise above these control mechanisms which really are out of date. The primate and primal instincts and reactions are no longer number one but quietly get regulated further and further into the background as the person emerges from the illusions of the life they had created.

For me writing this, many people in power will not like anything I am writing or saying. The pyramid of power is deeply embedded within humanity and those in control do not want you to become free from all of this. Many faiths, beliefs and religions will also not like any of this yet write and speak I must in an effort to help each of us and humanity.

As one practises Being Omni, these changes bring about freedom of the self from the self and you begin to enter a new state of interactiveness with all things. I call this commonalty: what is common for all people and for our place within this world.

Blank Spaces and Living Words

I read almost as much as I write and many, many books have helped and guided me on my journey of self-development and how to become me, from Richard Bach's *Jonathan Livingston Seagull* and *Illusions* and Paulo Coelho's books to Don Miguel Ruiz and *The Four Agreements.*

Sometimes I would run a talk or workshop and base them around books that I have read and that I think will help people. *Illusions* is a good example here. I would ask the students to read the book a few weeks before the course. When we met up I would ask them what is on the front cover? Even having just read the book, surprisingly very few could answer. I would ask other questions about the plot or characters much to the same effect. Thousands if not millions of people have read this book of self-help and freedom yet they miss so much because they are still stuck within the mind's views of their life so far.

There was also a discrepancy in what people had read. Take *The Pilgrimage* by Coelho. Many would read but not do the exercises. Many would read but not face their personal devil. Many would read but still never understand about love although clearly defined in the book.

So, what was the difference? I am the same as everyone else. Yet I seemed to find different messages within each book. And then I came across a quote by William Blake: "*Both read the Bible day and night, but thou read black where I read white.*" The last bit is the important bit ~ you read black while I read white. There is so much more than the written word...even the spaces mean something.

Another book by Coelho answered this. *The Witch of Portobello* is about a lady who learns how to master calligraphy. Her teacher waits until she can read and understand the spaces between each word where the writer's thoughts are hidden and where you can truly live and experience the book: "*And as you make those discoveries, you'll manage to fill in the blank spaces that all those writers left there on purpose to provoke the reader's imagination. And when you fill in the spaces, you'll start to believe in your own abilities.*"

In our haste to read, learn and pass the test, we glance over these spaces and so miss the chance to grow inside. It just becomes more knowledge to store. For many of these books, their meanings hit a spot within us and make us feel a little better but it is their simplicity that defeats us. We follow the story and feel better but never take the journey. Learn to live and experience a book or anything please.

It was this lesson, learning to read and experience the spaces in between, that helped me understand *living* words. It was not until my wife, Yvonne, placed *The Diary of a Magus* in front of me one day (because I was moaning that I had nothing to read), that I realised that it is not until you read the writing in living words that the book can really become lessons in self-discovery. This insight actually took me a while. The first time she gave this book to me, I dismissed it. A similar thing happened when Yvonne gave me the book *Ireland* by Frank Delaney as a Christmas present. I dismissed that one too. And yet both are life changing books when you read the writing in living words.

Most of us live a story, feeling the wind on our faces, experiencing the character's emotions and enjoying how the events of the story unfold. But even this level of engagement means it is still abstract to your life, separate from it so to speak. When read in living words, you immerse and live the moments in the story and your body flows with it too. I had the answer all the time to how I work, I just never realised that I too write in living words and speak at talks with words that are alive to that moment. I always want others to share what we are learning so would encourage this. But when other people reiterated them, they were lifeless and not animated. Their interpretations had gone via the mind so the words and meanings became conditioned and fixed. Not living at all.

Just as you learnt to read one syllable at a time which forms words, your mind begins to censor your input and we end up seeing only what the mind wants or allows us to see. This is why reading a self-help book more than once allows freedom within. As you practise Being Omni more and more, the mind's restrictions and limitations become greatly reduced, and the books reveal more and more.

So, we re-read and guess what? It's different this time. I did not see this or that last time I read. And each time they re-read the book, their eyes finally begin to open and their hearts enjoy a freedom from their mind.

Living words means that not only do enjoy the book you are reading but you begin to get a much deeper understanding of the story within, and also a shift within your consciousness happens which allows you to see clearly and perceive much more.

Further Reading

Jonathan Livingston Seagull – Richard Bach

This is a personal freedom book. It's all right not to fit and not to follow the crowd who have rules and regulations that you don't like.

It is a great little book that gives us a sense of freedom and adventure when we read it – far from the maddening crowd so to speak. It gives us hope and joy as long as we don't feel sorry for this outcast who is obsessed with flying faster and faster, even to his own demise. There is a streak of stubbornness in everyone, but most have an edge that stops them at the brink of danger...or change.

Illusions – Richard Bach

Another brilliant read and a great story, or is it? There is a grain of truth in most things we do or say or write. The best music, paintings and books are written from the writers' or artists' experiences or adventures in their lives. Most are conceived after an emotional set back and are the creator's responses to this. I believe everything in the book is possible: walking on water; sinking into the ground; not needing fuel for your vehicle and so on. But we have set limits to all the things we know or do. We *know* what will happen. We have set scenarios, which means that your car windscreen will be covered in flies or you will have to go to a petrol station, simply because that is what you believe and create for yourselves. Once you begin to explore and use Being Omni more and more, the limits you previously set diminish nicely.

My wife decided to start a little shop selling essential oils, crystals and gemstones and much more. It was a success and we had a treatment room where people could have reflexology and crystal healing and a few other things. After a while, people kept giving me copies of *Illusions* and I ended up with quite a few! I asked Yvonne why they were doing this. 'Just read the front cover,' she replied. Oh dear, this was something I did not want. But I have read the book many times now and it restores my faith in myself. And although I dwindle further and further away from people and their needs for someone to do magic or whatever, I do venture to teach them to do this for themselves.

We are all reluctant messiahs!

The Pilgrimage – Paulo Coelho

Coelho's first real book...or was it? The forerunner to this is *The Diary of a Magus* but *The Pilgrimage* was the one that became a best seller. Millions of people enjoyed the book and just like *Jonathan* it is linked to a sense of freedom and doing something and learning all at the same time. The book is inspirational and talks to all of us as we read and dream. Some actually planned to walk to Compostela and many actually did the walk but, sadly, Petrus is a one off! But if you do want to walk it and you are ready, a guide will appear. This is guaranteed but you have to be ready.

I live in a place where there are beaches, headlands and woodland walks on my doorstep. Often, while I am out and about, I will meet a guide (albeit unasked for), but a person will appear and walk a little with me and, during that time, a lesson happens. Sometimes a lesson begins and the guide has vanished before I understand it so then I forget it or let it go, as a good Omni person should do. But guess what? The guide reappears and second or final part of the lesson happens. There is just no escaping sometimes when life is trying to teach you something!

Please note that this is not unique to me, it happens for every one. Absolutely true.

Every single day, lessons are there. It does not matter what your circumstances are. Imagine a person who is in prison and locked away in solitary confinement where there are no guides or teachers and very little external contact. One day an awakening happens within and a realisation that I am not an animal, I am Robert – a shift and a change has occurred and Robert no longer fits in a cage. Externally, the guards seem to know this. It may be days or weeks but as long as Robert maintains the shift, he will be let out of solitary. And as long as that change of state continues, he will become a free man. He may still be a criminal or, in my terms, a bit wayward but he will never go back to prison. I have Doug Hooper's, *You Are What You Think*, to thank for that lesson.

The Pilgrimage is an inspirational book that guides you from a distance and, in doing so, it opens the door for you to begin your lessons.

The reason you miss these opportunities and lessons is because you are just not present. Full stop. You may think you are but use Step Three and find your true answer please.

The Alchemist – Paulo Coelho

An all-time favourite. The main character, Santiago, goes on a journey with ups and downs and highs and lows. It is an adventure that allows the magic to flow and journeys across continents. It is rich with individual stories of the people he meets along the way. From the crystal merchant who too understands omens to the Englishman with a never-ending thirst for more knowledge from the books written by those who never succeed no matter what their writings proclaim.

It all begins because Santiago has a dream. A dream his parents, who are stuck forever within a harsh existence, give their blessing to even though they give away their one chance of freedom. Each encounter Santiago has speaks volumes so you can learn the lessons from the book without ever having to leave your armchair. It also teaches simple alchemy but few ever realise or practise these humble skills. The magic of *just being you* happens to Santiago many times. Love for Fatima, a woman of the desert, enables him to overcome need and greed. But gold and fortune await you too and at no cost either. Gosh, what a book to set us free... ah, but does the mind have the last say?

The world of books is ever a lie but there are hints and truths within them all. The alchemist in the story does exist eternally within the desert of his soul and very often he is out and about around your neighbourhood too!

The Four Agreements – Don Miguel Ruiz

An incredible book and a real life-changer for so many. It inspires us, corrects us, helps us help ourselves but very few pass the tests within the book. It is a book that you read and then must implement for yourself on a minute-by-minute basis. You must take Ruiz's words and make them your own, please. The four agreements really do work when you use and apply them to your life and the way you live.

But to really move on, you have to understand the first part of the book: human domestication and then self-domestication (your own domestication). We have wrongly learnt that to be in a group of like-minded people who suffer the same things, helps in some way. No. It only cements the problems and can even worsen them too. The agreements will work if used in the right ways. Freedom of domestication beckons but does require effort.

Also, learn to create some of your own personal, on-the-spot agreements. Learn to forgive and forget from a personal viewpoint. Many people carry scars of incidents and events that happen to them and even years later the scar may burn you again. Events often recycle themselves in our lives; some may say it's a lesson to learn. Omni people do not think this – something happens, they react then reset and move on which leaves no scars. The longer you stay angry at someone or something that happens, the deeper the scar and the greater the risk of illness. Your choice from now on.

Jacob the Baker – Noah benShea

A wonderful read that lifts and lightens us exponentially. It is so simple and enjoyable to read with such great wisdom and lessons contained within. It also helps us to feel good and just but this fades as with many books. Please persevere with it to learn to understand Jacob himself and his story as it helps you become you in small but lasting ways. Remember the pigeons know no better than the people expecting wisdoms and solutions from Jacob.

*****

There are so many books that have helped me along the path and I would be here for ever writing about them. They all help once you can read them with the right eyes and ears and are free of the mind's censorship which is worse than any computer spyware.

The books do help with some inspiration along the way but when you use the Omni steps often enough, the lessons happen and are easy to complete.

Stop and remember: Being Omni is the greatest shortcut to being you without any baggage.

Times, consciousness, lives and the world have changed. Life for many has become hard, and it does not matter what we know or what we have learnt or even believe in, it is not really helping people. So many are struggling to survive and even if you have therapy or counselling, it only helps short term.

Omni counselling is really simple ~ you start by doing and using the three, basic Omni steps. And breathe...

Good luck, (oops that's not the Omni way!)

Robert and Heather

A final note

How Omni has come about

It was early in 2014, at a talk in Cirencester, that Omni came to the forefront of things. Although, for many years, I have been using the words *Omni presence* to describe a state of being that helps all people. But at that time, it became the word Omni ~ it stood alone and perfect with its own resonance.

Many months passed and I had almost forgotten about it, until one morning, while on my usual walk along the beach with the dogs, I kept hearing the word, Omni. It was persistent and kept getting louder as I walked towards the headland. I kept saying I would deal with it later on, but it got louder and eventually the headland shook a little with its resonance. *Okay*, I said and confirmed I would write about it in the afternoon. This was still not good enough, it has to be written about now! So, I said that I would. And a great sigh went out into the universe and the old gods, avatars, plus plenty whose time had come years before, were released and free.

This all sounds a little grand and even biblical and I am not one for listening to spirits or gods but nevertheless, it did happen.

I came home from my walk and created the Omni page and began to put a few words on it. A friend of mine said about experiencing a strange but good energy shift and going into a state of being that she was not used to or experienced before. It seemed that Omni was working with or without me.

But we have a propensity to seek out all about something, to define it and to label it and, ultimately, this destroys it. I believe Omni can evade this because it is undefinable. It is simply a way to for you to be. The duality within will deny it. We are human beings with all sorts of good and bad things about each of us, yet we were sent down a false trail of having to be good because of belief systems. We end up crucifying ourselves by having to be something we are not. Once you are used to Being Omni there is no right or wrong, even love is blind to it.

For millions and millions of people who are believers in religions, Omni is an anathema because it does not rely on any external beliefs. Its only belief is self-belief and better still, belief in the self ~ YOU. Anyone can utilise the steps and also maintain their faiths and beliefs and still grow.

Humanity, despite all its growth, has forgotten how to look after itself. Many people suffer with stress, anxiety, depression and many other mind-orientated illnesses: Omni puts people first in the simplest of ways. When a person begins to use Being Omni and can keep up this practice then they benefit and all that they know can share these benefits.

Life is all about stages and these determine different times and ages of our lives. Being Omni is just the first stage of your journey and once there is a sense of these steps becoming a more natural part of your everyday life, there is a point where you shift into Omni Being. But please remember, experience then let go of it.

The point of power is only ever in the nows and moments.

∞

Bibliography

Bach, R (2003), *Jonathan Livingston Seagull,* London: Harper Element

Bach, R (1992), *Illusions*, London: Arrow Books

benShea, N (1989), *Jacob the Baker*, USA: Ballantine Books

Coelho, P (2009), *The Witch of Portobello*, London: HarperCollins

Coelho, P (1992), *The Diary of a Magus*, NY, America: HarperCollins

Coelho, P (1997), *The Alchemist*, London: Thorsons

Coelho, P (2003), *The Pilgrimage*, London: Harper

Delaney, F (2004), *Ireland*, London, UK: Time Warner Books

Dwyer, W (2001), *10 Secrets for Success and Inner Peace*, United States of America, Australia, UK, South Africa, India and Canada: Hay House Inc.

Haye, L (1984), *You Can Heal Your Life*, United States of America, Australia, UK, South Africa, India and Canada: Hay House Inc.

Hooper, D (1992), *You Are What You Think*, New York, USA: Prentice Hall

Ruiz, D M (1997) *The Four Agreements*, San Rafael, California: Amber-Allen

Tolle, E (2005), *The Power of Now*, London: Hodder and Stoughton

Wilde, S (1996), *Silent Power*, California, USA: Hay House Inc.